Praise 1

"In my practice, we check the testosterone levels of all men over the age of thirty-five who feel depressed. We do this before we discuss antidepression medications or engage in a course of talk therapy. Checking their testosterone is the starting point.

The power of Dr. Maupin and Mr. Newcomb's approach is that it offers science-based medicine and is psychologically sound, all in one package. It's often difficult to find the former in the average low-T clinic; it's unheard of to find the latter. This is pioneering work, and mainstream medicine will be following their lead."

— Michael E. Mahon, PsyD
Saint Louis, Missouri

"As both trailblazers and advocates for women's health, Dr. Kathy Maupin and Brett Newcomb let the secret out when they revealed the absolute importance testosterone plays in promoting the health and well-being of women in their first book, *The Secret Female Hormone*. Applying the training and education received at Dr. Maupin's clinic in St. Louis using the pellet method for bioidentical hormone replacement, the female patients seen in our clinic experience a higher quality of life, better health, and a restored personal sense of well-being. As a result, many of them ask, "What can I do to get my husband to come see you?" The answer is now quite simple: Have him read this book and let's see what happens! I am grateful for this important resource that emphasizes the crucial role testosterone plays in men's health."

— Jason M. Kolodjski, DC, MSN, APRN, FNP-C
Clinic Director, Natural Health Center
Houston, Texas

GOT TESTOSTERONE?™

Men—Return to the Sexier, Smarter, Stronger You!

By Kathy Maupin, MD
and Brett Newcomb, MA, LPC

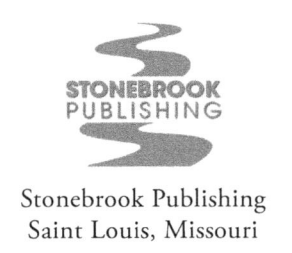

Stonebrook Publishing
Saint Louis, Missouri

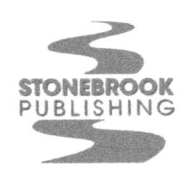

A STONEBROOK PUBLISHING BOOK

Copyright © 2019 by Kathy Maupin, MD

This book was guided in development and edited by
Nancy Erickson, The Book Professor®
TheBookProfessor.com

All rights reserved. Published in the United States by Stonebrook Publishing, a division of Stonebrook Enterprises, LLC, Saint Louis, Missouri. No part of this book may be reproduced, scanned, or distributed in any printed or electronic form without written permission from the author.

Please do not participate in or encourage piracy of copyrighted materials in violation of the author's rights.

Library of Congress Control Number: 2018963789

ISBN: 978-1-7322767-5-8

www.stonebrookpublishing.net

PRINTED IN THE UNITED STATES OF AMERICA

10 9 8 7 6 5 4 3 2 1

Dedication

This book is dedicated to men everywhere who are fighting the battle against aging and are looking for affordable, practical answers in their quest to remain vigorous and healthy for the rest of their lives.

We wrote this book to provide answers to those challenges. We didn't write it for young weight-lifter men who want to bulk up. It's not meant to turn you into a muscle-bound, no-neck caricature of masculinity, although this book will help you maintain your muscle mass. It wasn't written to make you hypersexual, although the solution found within will help you be sexual and have a strong libido. Neither is it for medicating you, although it will help you avoid the need for certain meds that are associated with aging and will prevent you from ever needing many of them.

This book was written with respect and careful detail, and it tells the stories of real men who have overcome many of the difficulties and diseases of aging by accepting the optimal testosterone replacement.

To my patients who may identify with one or more of the "real life" examples in this book, I assure you that I have combined several case studies into each example, so no person will feel that I have revealed their secrets.

My hope is that you and the next generation of men over forty will maintain your strength, sexuality, and confidence—as well as your good health—for the rest of your life.

Contents

Foreword by John Maupin, JD xiii

Preface xv

Acknowledgments xix

Chapter 1: The One Hormone Men Need to Sustain Their Youth and Health 1

Chapter 2: Do You Have Any of the Symptoms of Low Testosterone?. 11
    Erectile Dysfunction 16
    Infrequent or Decreased Volume of Ejaculation. 21
    Loss of Sexual Desire 22
    Inability to Achieve an Orgasm. 25
    Premature Ejaculation 27
    Loss of Morning Erections. 27
    Loss of Muscle Mass. 29
    Loss of Stamina and Strength. 33
    Poor Recovery After a Heart Attack. 34
    Insomnia / Poor Quality Sleep 35
    Fatigue 38
    Memory Problems 41

Joint Aches / Arthritis *43*
Poor Balance / Coordination *44*
The All-American Beer Belly *46*
Ringing in the Ears *47*
Anxiety and Depression *47*
Man Boobs *51*
Smaller Genitals *52*
Feeling Old and Near the End of Life *54*
More Body Hair but Less Head Hair *55*
New Migraine Headaches *56*
Thinning Skin *58*
Frequent Urination / Enlarged Prostate *59*

Chapter 3: Do You Have Any of the Diseases or Conditions of Aging? Testosterone Can Help! 63
Insulin Resistance *68*
Adult-Onset Diabetes *69*
Obesity *71*
High Cholesterol, Triglycerides, and Inflammation *73*
Parkinson's Disease *74*
Osteoporosis *77*
Autoimmune Diseases: Rheumatoid Arthritis, Systemic Lupus, Crohn's Disease, Multiple Sclerosis, Scleroderma, Psoriasis, and Fibromyalgia *81*
Dementia and Alzheimer's Disease *83*
Male Breast Cancer *89*
Cancer *90*
Sarcopenia *91*
Risk of Early Mortality *93*

Chapter 4: Testosterone Pellets: The Best Option for Men 95
 How Do the Ease of Treatment and the Cost of Different Forms of Testosterone Compare? *96*
 How Do the Medical Benefits and Risks of Different Forms of Testosterone Compare? *99*
 Testosterone Gel: The Most Common Testosterone Replacement *101*
 Potential Side Effects of Testosterone Replacement *103*
 Conversions into Estrogens *103*
 Unfounded Concern About Prostate Cancer and Testosterone *105*

Chapter 5: Interpreting Your Blood Tests 109
 Preparing for Your Blood Tests *110*
 Interpreting Your Blood Tests *111*
 Panel of Blood Tests *112*
 Abnormal Blood Tests That Could Prevent You From Receiving T Pellets *114*
 Explanation of and Treatment for Abnormal Blood Labs *114*
 Testing of Hormones from Non-Sex Glands in the Body: Cortisol, Thyroid, T3, T4, Reverse T3 . . . . *120*
 Blood Tests That Reflect Your Cardiac Health *123*
 Blood Tests That Reflect Your General Health *126*
 Cancer Screening Tests *130*
 The Art and Science of Laboratory Interpretation *131*

Chapter 6: Sex and Testosterone: How It Works and What Can Go Wrong 133
 Biological and Physical Issues *133*
 Relationship Issues *158*

Chapter 7: Special Circumstances and Treatments 177
    When a Man Is Not Yet Ready for Testosterone Pellets 177
    When Testosterone Pellets Aren't an Option. 186

Conclusion 189

Appendix A: Questions Men Ask 193
    The Superiority of Testosterone Pellets 193
    Testosterone and Erectile Dysfunction. 198
    Testosterone and Prostate Cancer. 200
    Other Aspects of Testosterone 202
    Your Lifestyle: How It Affects the Success of T Pellet Treatment. 203
    How T Pellets Influence the Diseases of Aging 203
    Side Effects of Testosterone Pellets. 205

Appendix B: Hormone Imbalances That Cause Symptoms of Aging. 209

Appendix C: Dr. Maupin's Low-Carb Diet for Men 211

Appendix D: How to Make Sure Your PSA Test Is Accurate. 215

About the Authors 217
    Kathy Maupin, MD 217
    Brett Newcomb, MA, LPC 218

Foreword

Right off the bat, you should know that I'm Dr. Kathy Maupin's husband of forty-plus years. Kathy and I got married after her first year of medical school, so I was along for the ride, practicing law as she worked hard and progressed to become a board-certified OB/GYN.

As Kathy's career unfolded, I also witnessed her struggle to find a way to provide her patients with a better quality of life as they aged. Because her patients were exclusively female, her sole focus was on women, and she accomplished her goal as evidenced by her first book with Brett Newcomb, *The Secret Female Hormone: How Testosterone Replacement Can Change Your Life*, published in six countries on four continents.

The success with her female patients led to an unexpected problem: the husbands couldn't keep up with their revitalized wives. So, many of Kathy's patients asked if she would treat their husbands. She was initially reluctant, not because the science of male hormonal therapy was foreign to her, but because she thought men already had good options. Then Kathy investigated those other treatment regimens and discovered they were far from satisfactory and, in fact, were sometimes dangerous. Most had very little physician oversight and took the one-size-fits-all approach, which rarely works for hormone replacement.

So Kathy did for men what she had previously done for women—she developed an individualized treatment protocol based on each patient's thorough medical history and a complete workup using specific blood tests. By using very small pellets of bioidentical testosterone that are placed under the skin, she has been able to restore much of the vitality that her male patients enjoyed in their prime.

I became one of Kathy's first patients and can attest to a renewal of energy, muscle tone, and overall good health. I lost weight and became leaner, and my hereditary high blood pressure and high cholesterol required far less medication.

Many of my friends have been curious about the treatment. I tell them the insertions are virtually painless and last four to six months. The treatment plan addresses far more than simply erectile dysfunction, and the benefits extend far beyond the bedroom. Of course, Kathy doesn't tell me who her patients are, but that doesn't stop *them* from telling *me* how BioBalance Health® has changed their lives. They are thrilled and happy to spread the word.

This book contains detailed information about testosterone hormone replacement therapy for men, set forth in a nonscientific style that allows you to discover if it could be right for you. It presents the medical situations of actual patients, showing how Kathy and her medical team assess and treat a wide range of conditions with pellet therapy and other useful alternatives.

I look forward to a long and healthy life filled with travel, golf, a new granddaughter, and all the good things that go along with them. I hope you, too, will consider bioidentical testosterone pellet therapy to enhance your life.

John Maupin, JD

Preface

After the publication of our first book, *The Secret Female Hormone: How Testosterone Replacement Can Change Your Life*, Brett Newcomb and I were frequently asked, "When are you going to write a book about testosterone pellets for men?"

I was initially reluctant to take on such a task for two reasons. First, I was trained as an OB/GYN, and my treatment of men had originally been limited to their infertility issues. When I was in medical school in the 1970s, I made a conscious decision to exclusively treat women because, frankly, male patients in that era wouldn't listen to a female doctor. But this present generation of men is quite different, and they often prefer female physicians over male doctors. My second reason for shying away from a book about testosterone for men was that mainstream medicine was already offering men many alternatives for testosterone treatment, and they didn't seem to need any more direction.

Both of those preconceived notions were incorrect. I started treating men when my rejuvenated female patients asked me to help their husbands get "back in the game." These women wanted me to treat their husbands with the same bioidentical testosterone pellets that they themselves had received because they felt so re-enlivened. Soon, the BioBalance® method of replacing men's testosterone using pellets gave them fuller and more robust lives, and the men were enthusiastic about their treatment and the results they'd achieved. I realized I'd found an effective and superior testosterone replacement for men and was inspired to write a book to answer the questions men have about testosterone replacement.

Most of my male patients had tried some other testosterone or ED treatment before they came to me. I quickly learned that these other treatments were frequently substandard in every respect except cost. Then I started paying greater attention to the advertising for these men's clinics and observed that the approaches often were dangerously deficient in one or more ways, the information they presented to their patients was simply wrong, and finally, most of them didn't use testosterone pellets. Of course, the men had no way of knowing any of this because there was no easy reference source for them.

Consequently, I recruited Brett Newcomb to work with me to write a second book about testosterone, this time aimed at a male audience. I had to continue my life's mission of helping my patients and others live their lives to their fullest, and that meant reaching out to men.

This book addresses the questions I answer on a daily basis about what we do at BioBalance Health®, why we employ the protocols we use, how we screen patients to identify those whom we can help, and why our approach is superior to others.

This book contains real-life scenarios based on conditions I've treated. None of the stories are about specific patients; just the variety of situations I've encountered. So if a story seems personally familiar, don't worry! It's not about you. Readers have told us they like this approach because, from these stories, they see that they're not alone. Others have had the same problems and challenges and have overcome them. As I tell my shy patients, "Don't worry. You can't tell me anything I haven't heard before."

After a full assessment of a man's bloodwork and medical history to determine if he'll respond well to our treatment, we administer bioidentical testosterone pellets that are made from yams and compounded by trusted pharmacists. The pellets are inserted beneath a man's skin two or three times a year, depending on his metabolism. This is by far the most convenient, reliable, and effective treatment available anywhere today.

In this book, we also relied on Brett's decades of experience in counseling to expand the discussion beyond the medical issues and address the relational challenges that are often present in the male-female dynamic. Sorry to disappoint some of you, but the largest sex organ in humans is the *brain*! And that's why Brett's insights are very helpful—and often transformational.

You don't have to succumb to the diseases of aging or live the miserable life of an aging, impotent, frail old man. Testosterone pellets can change your life, as you'll read in the pages that follow.

Kathy Maupin, MD
Founder and Medical Director
BioBalance Health® LLC
Saint Louis, Missouri

Acknowledgments

We want to express our deep and profound appreciation for the support and help we received while writing this book from our spouses, John Maupin and Phyllis Newcomb. Without their encouragement, editing, and creative support, we could never have accomplished anything as significant as a book. Their help with topics for the health podcasts we produce, their encouragement for the segments of the book that they read, and their suggestions for the phrasing and organization of our manuscript were invaluable.

We also owe an enormous debt to Joe Baalman, the COO of BioBalance Health® and BioBalance Skin®. Joe is our cameraman, our film editor, and our graphics designer, as well as our reliable anchor for keeping the businesses going while we work on learning more about hormones and the treatments we describe in this book.

As we've learned more about hormone treatments, particularly for men, we've come to rely on the contributions of Dr. Rachel Maupin Sullivan, a partner at BioBalance Health® and BioBalance Skin®. She has a driving intellect and a passionate investment in helping us learn the newest and most reliable information about changes in the thinking and practice of hormone treatments for men.

We want to express our appreciation to the BioBalance staff for their professionalism and their encouragement and support.

And finally, we want to thank our editor/publisher Nancy Erickson, The Book Professor®. Without her organizational skills and her suggestions for the content and structure of our writing, this book would never have materialized.

CHAPTER 1

The One Hormone Men Need to Sustain Their Youth and Health

If your doctor asked you the following question, how would you respond? "If I prescribed just one hormone that would keep you healthy, strong, and fully productive from today until right before you die, would you take it?"

You might jump at the opportunity and say "yes" right away, feeling thrilled that one simple treatment could take care of many of your physical ills for the rest of your life. But it's more likely that you'd ask a lot of reasonable questions before you considered this a good option, such as:

- Is it affordable? *Yes!*
- Are there many side effects? *No!*
- Is it difficult to follow the directions? *No! Simply visit the doctor two or three times a year.*
- Will I lose any of my current skills or brain power? *No!*
- Does it really work? *Yes!*

These questions are valid and should be asked about any medical treatment that sounds too good to be true. And after seeing the answers, you might have enough information to act.

Or perhaps not. You might have some more personal questions for a physician like me, such as:

- Would you or do you take this hormone? *Absolutely! I have taken it for the last fifteen years.*
- Would you prescribe it to your husband? *Yes! He has taken it for twelve years.*
- Are you healthier now than you were when you were younger—before you started this medication? *I am, and I can't imagine that I'd be working or having any fun at all if I hadn't started taking this hormone!*

Testosterone, in bioidentical form, has been hidden away in the structure of yams since they were first cultivated. It was discovered that yams contain testosterone, and the hormone is extracted in a laboratory using specific chemicals that separate the "wheat from the chaff," so to speak, eliminating everything except the testosterone. The testosterone is then compounded into time-release pellets that are inserted in a man's buttocks or love handles.

Testosterone, in bioidentical form, has been hidden away in the structure of yams since they were first cultivated.

Ever since medical school, I've been searching for the single source of the diseases of aging and its associated disabilities. I spent a lot of time at the University of Missouri School of Medicine and at the Veterans Administration Hospital and couldn't bear to tell my patients that they simply had to accept the fact that they could no longer walk, or drive, or stand up simply because they were *old*.

I couldn't find an answer for the infirmities of aging through pharmacology, and so I began looking for a remedy at the beginning stages of life. I specialized as an OB/GYN, hoping to make pregnant women the healthiest incubators for human life as possible. That work, I thought, would produce healthier children, who would one day age in a healthier manner. But after years of delivering babies, I realized that while I might have helped deliver healthier children through excellent prenatal care, when they turned forty, they still seemed to crash!

That's exactly what happened to me at age forty. I started experiencing things I never had before: fatigue, migraines, and depression. I was cranky and irritable at home; working thirty-six hour shifts as an OB/GYN was nearly impossible. But I had to plunge ahead because I had no other options and there was no cure.

By the time I was forty-seven, I could still work, but I had crippling pain from endometriosis, a disease of the ovaries for which surgery is the only curative treatment. Thinking that my ovaries were the source of my misery, I had a hysterctomy. But I had an unusual complication and after surgery, I ended up on a respirator in the ICU. While I was there, I had a near-death experience. In other words, I died in the ICU but was brought back to life. I came back from death certain that God had given me a mission, although I didn't yet know what it was.

The six months after my hysterectomy were the worst of my life. I was even more fatigued and depressed, and I had daily migraines that incapacitated me. Why on earth had I been brought back? Why hadn't I been allowed to die? What good could I possibly do if I couldn't work anymore? I sought help from dozens of doctors, but they all told me to "just live with it." I gained twenty pounds and, emotionally, I gave up.

There is great power in giving over to God what you can't do yourself, and when I did that, I got an immediate answer to my health crisis. I was introduced to the doctor who saved my life—with testosterone pellets. Dr. Gino Tutera instantly knew what was wrong with me: I had no testosterone. He treated me with estradiol and testosterone pellets, and I immediately started to get better.

I discovered my new calling: help other women who had found no relief from their debilitation symptoms of menopause. The answer was to replace their lost testosterone using compounded pellets made of bioidentical testosterone extracted from yams. It came to me at the perfect time and place, as it often is with those who trust in God. I'd finally found the answer to the question I'd had in medical school: What's the one thing that triggers the disease of aging, and how can we treat it? Testosterone!

> **In reality, aging isn't an inevitable process without a cause—or thousands of causes. It begins with testosterone loss and is treated with testosterone pellets.**

In reality, aging isn't an inevitable process without a cause—or thousands of causes. It begins with testosterone loss and is treated with testosterone pellets.

Soon my women patients begged me to treat their husbands like I had treated them. I was trained to do so, but I hadn't taken care of men since I did infertility work early in my practice. Today, treating men is the fastest-growing part of my practice.

Aging EQUALS Testosterone Deficiency Syndrome (TDS)

"You don't have low testosterone. You're just getting old, and you'll have to live with it!"

Thousands of times per day, men are told that they don't have low testosterone when they may or may not have been tested for *total* and *free* testosterone. This "medical" advice is categorically wrong! Aging and TDS go hand in hand, and the syndromes can be reversed with the proper testosterone replacement. If you've received this kind of advice, please find a new doctor!

The truth is that aging and testosterone deficiency are one and the same. What society views as the effects of aging—lack of libido, weight gain, belly fat, man boobs, fatigue, lack of motivation, and a slow, stooped gate—are not inevitable. They are characteristics of aging that can be reversed if treated with testosterone replacement before severe physical changes have occurred.

The most important thing to remember is this: whether you've tried testosterone replacement or not, it's critically important to receive the safest, most effective testosterone treatment before you give up on yourself and decide that you're doomed to live with the ravages of aging. Sadly, both men and women have been convinced they can do nothing about the symptoms of aging that drain them of vitality year after year, but it's simply not true.

> **The truth is that aging and testosterone deficiency are one and the same.**

Diagnosing TDS: Blood Hormone Levels and Symptoms

When you go to your doctor to inquire whether your symptoms are those of TDS, your doctor should order blood tests. He or she should be looking for *specific data points* from your blood chemistry that indicate testosterone deficiency.

The following is a bit technical, but it's important. If your blood hormone level of total testosterone is below 400 nanograms per deciliter, and your free testosterone is below 129 pg/ml, then you have blood levels that qualify you to be diagnosed with TDS.

Less important but other informative blood levels include LH (lutenizing hormone), estrone, and DHT (dihydrotestosterone). If LH is low, then you have TDS from pituitary insufficiency; or if LH is above 8, you have testicular failure. Testosterone replacement can be used to treat both conditions.

Estrone blood levels above 30 pg/ml indicate a high estrogen that binds up testosterone and makes it inactive. Lastly, if DHT, a by-product of testosterone, is less than 25, a low free testosterone blood level is confirmed. The second part of the qualifications that diagnose TDS include the symptoms discussed in chapter 2

If you have the symptoms of TDS that are outlined in chapter 2 and have a total T level less than 400 in the morning—or a free T level less than 129—you should consider testosterone replacement. As a comparison, when you are young and healthy, your levels should range between 400 and 1,500 nanograms per deciliter (ng/dl) of testosterone. The goal is to restore you to a young man's healthy level.

Do *YOU* Have TDS?

The first step to determine if you have TDS is to carefully review each of the symptoms of testosterone deficiency syndrome described in chapter 2. Ask yourself these questions:

- Is this me?
- Do I feel like this?
- Is this how I feel when I think to myself, *I'm just getting old!*

In general, men aren't as introspective as women, so they leave it to their female friends or spouses to observe and inform them about the changes they see. If you have one of those females watching over you, then let them help you answer the questions that may lead you to a whole new life!

Shortly after I was married forty years ago, I studied my husband's morning routine at the sink. First, he tried to pry his eyes open; then he splashed water on his face; then he applied shaving cream and scraped away the previous day's bristle. And after he had done all this, he did the most curious thing: he leaned into the mirror, smiled at himself, tried on some facial expressions that showed deep appreciation for what he saw, and then he raised both arms up like Rocky and rotated in front of the mirror and stated, "I look great, don't I!"

What self-esteem, what beautiful, unabashed admiration he had for his male form! I had *never* felt like that when looking in the mirror, and I dare say most women don't. We pick at ourselves, find the most hated part of our face or body, and then worry over it all day. How I admired his male confidence!

One of the reasons that men have such natural self-satisfaction is their high level of testosterone. It's all based on the hormones that bathe the brain.

Perhaps you're nodding and you agree that you like what you see in the mirror—or at least you remember when you did.

But most men start to feel the stab of self-doubt when they watch their flat stomach turn into a beer belly and they see their forehead grow. Men don't become insecure because they think they're changing from handsome to ugly. They become insecure because, as the level of free testosterone drops and physical changes make aging more evident, they no longer have the "juice" that gives them confidence and allows them to appreciate their own physical attributes.

Relationship Consequences of TDS

We humans seem to deny any symptoms of illness until we've become overwhelmed by them or fear that we're dying. Therefore, sexual dysfunction is generally ignored or is blamed on other life events, such as having young children in the house or fighting with a spouse. Or, worse, you ignore sexual dysfunction because your doctor says your testosterone levels test normal and you should "just take this blue pill before sex."

This book was written to reach men while they're early in the process and still in the "loss of libido" stage; that is, before they experience dysfunction and disease. The motivation is *prevention*— to prevent the *relationship issues* that inevitably follow loss of libido and onset of ED and to prevent the *medical problems* that are secondary to TDS, specifically, erectile dysfunction, diabetes, hypertension, and heart disease.

When TDS is not recognized for what it is, marriages and intimate partnerships suffer. Without proper diagnosis, partners notice the man's loss of desire and often think it's because their partner's feelings about them have changed. They may think that their partner has found another love interest or that there's something about *them* that repels. (See more in the second part of chapter 2.)

When TDS is not recognized for what it is, marriages and intimate partnerships suffer.

If men can't discuss the changes they're experiencing openly and honestly, then their relationship with their partner becomes a rollercoaster of emotional turmoil. They are often accused of infidelity. Sometimes their partners seek other sources of affection to either reassure *them* that they're still attractive or to maintain their own sense of emotional security.

Although it's a skill that many men haven't developed, being able to communicate about the perceived change in their libido and what it might mean is very important. The absence of clear communication leads to frustrated relationships. Without this emotional awareness and sensitivity to his partner, a man can't reassure his partner that he still loves her and needs her. Thus, he is withholding something that she fundamentally needs.

Sexual symptoms of TDS include the loss of morning erections, infrequent or absent ejaculation, reduced penis size, and a decrease in frequency and sustained erections. Other causes for these symptoms must also be considered, but in a significant portion of the male population, these symptoms indicate TDS.

There are other symptoms that are signs of TDS, including insomnia and fatigue. A man will begin to recognize that his body won't do what he's always expected it to do. He'll tire more readily and won't sleep as well.

In addition to fatigue and insomnia, many men experience a loss of motivation—their "get up and go" seems to have gotten up and gone. They begin to notice memory problems, such as not being able to recall the name of someone they know well, or they have a sense of grasping for a word that they know, but it won't appear when they want to use it. They may begin to have migraine headaches and joint aches or what they believe is arthritis, and they may experience poor balance or coordination. Other symptoms include decreased muscle mass and strength. They can no longer restore their muscle mass through exercise alone. And then there's the belly fat and "man boobs." If these symptoms are familiar to you, you've probably got TDS.

There are also emotional effects of TDS. Men who experience all or many of these symptoms may also begin to suffer from depression and anxiety attacks. Anxiety attacks begin even when their stress levels have not changed much and their relationships are stable. If a man then receives a drug to fight depression, his depression often gets much worse. We have found that depression and anxiety that begins after age forty is often successfully treated with testosterone and does not require psychiatric drugs.

As men age, they need to redefine their sense of self. When they reach retirement age, they have to rediscover who they are and how they define and experience themselves. The pain and process of rediscovery is compounded if they are suffering from TDS. The process is difficult enough as it is, but it doesn't have to be compounded by undiagnosed and untreated low testosterone levels.

The best remedy to the relationship issues and physical symptoms of TDS is to replace lost testosterone by using long-acting bioidentical testosterone pellets. I've used all forms of testosterone replacement therapies, and patients treated with other types of testosterone and the associated delivery methods have been overwhelmingly disappointed. Bioidentical testosterone pellets are the only form of testosterone that satisfy.

The best remedy to the relationship issues and physical symptoms of TDS is to replace lost testosterone by using long-acting bioidentical testosterone pellets.

The purpose of this book to explain to men that what they have always believed about getting old is *not* true; that there is an affordable, effective, and safe treatment to help them avoid what has always been accepted as destiny; that getting old and sick is not inevitable if they replace their testosterone in the safest and most natural way, through testosterone pellets.

Men, you now have the power to change the second half century of your life. My hope is that you and the next generation of men over forty will maintain your strength, sexuality, and confidence, as well as your good health, for all of your life.

What You Get When You've "Got Testosterone" with T Pellets

Isn't the chance to realize these benefits worth your time to investigate if you have TDS and, if so, taking the step to raise your testosterone level with T pellets:

- Long, productive life
- Improved quality of life
- Great sex life and improved partner relationships
- Lower costs for your future medical care
- Delaying the need to live in an "old folk's home"
- Ability to work and play longer
- Fewer doctor visits, injuries, and surgeries
- Fewer prescription medications
- Ability to exercise for the rest of your life

CHAPTER 2

Do You Have Any of the Symptoms of Low Testosterone?

Symptoms of Testosterone Deficiency in Men

- ❏ Erectile Dysfunction
- ❏ Infrequent or Decreased Volume of Ejaculation
- ❏ Loss of Sexual Desire
- ❏ Inability to Achieve an Orgasm
- ❏ Premature Ejaculation
- ❏ Loss of Morning Erections
- ❏ Loss of Muscle Mass
- ❏ Loss of Stamina and Strength
- ❏ Poor Recovery After a Heart Attack
- ❏ Insomnia/ Poor Quality Sleep
- ❏ Fatigue
- ❏ Memory Problems from Low Testosterone
- ❏ Joint Aches / Arthritis

- ❑ Poor Balance / Coordination
- ❑ The All-American Beer Belly
- ❑ Ringing in the Ears
- ❑ Anxiety and Depression
- ❑ Man Boobs
- ❑ Smaller Genitals
- ❑ Feeling Old and Near the End of Life
- ❑ More Body Hair but Less Head Hair
- ❑ New Migraine Headaches
- ❑ Thinning Skin
- ❑ Frequent Urination / Enlarged Prostate

Testosterone deficiency syndrome (TDS) is *real*, and all men with three or more of the symptoms listed above should not request, but demand, an evaluation for low testosterone by their family doctor, urologist, or testosterone hormone replacement specialist. The diagnosis of TDS, followed by treatment with the proper testosterone pellet formulation, will literally *save* your life, not just make it better! While it's true that most kinds of testosterone will improve your sex life, only testosterone pellets improve *everything*: your life, health, and sex.

The lack of testosterone, or TDS, as shown above, causes a long list of symptoms that can lead to many diseases of aging. Acknowledging that you have many of these symptoms is your first step to getting your life back. It's vital for you to carefully consider whether you have any of the symptoms we describe in this chapter. If you have more than three of them, you may be suffering from TDS.

Some men are bothered that they can't do the things they did just a few years ago, such as snow ski, swim laps, or walk more than a few blocks without becoming breathless. If that sounds familiar, you should stop and ask yourself, "Why?" The symptoms of TDS can creep up on a man so slowly that he doesn't see the pattern until he reviews a full list of symptoms and checks off each one he has. When you acknowledge the symptoms in yourself, it's the first step to getting your life back.

This book provides you with the tools you need to diagnose *yourself* because many doctors are clueless about how important it is to treat TDS. When asked about it, most of them just shrug and tell you that you're simply getting older. Please do not accept this opinion without having your blood drawn and evaluated by an expert physician who understands TDS (see more in chapter 4). Sadly, complaints about the symptoms of aging are frequently ignored rather than diagnosed and treated as low testosterone.

Many doctors—and remember that I am one—like to offer a bit of paternalistic BS to ease their day and stay on their office schedule. If what you have isn't life-threatening, then doctors could deem it unimportant and not worthy of their time. A little thing like your marriage or your satisfaction with life is not "their problem," or so all doctors were trained to believe thirty or more years ago. Therefore, doctors are trained to bully you into accepting your disability and illness of TDS by telling you the symptoms are normal aging and there's nothing you can do about it. In my opinion, declaring that men as young as forty years old have "old age" commits them to spending half their life hurting, sleepless, weak, and sexless. That sounds like a terminal disease to me, but it's usually accepted or ignored by mainstream doctors.

The most compassionate doctors may offer a simple one-pill-answer to a man's complaints about sexual dysfunction—Viagra® or Cialis®. But just because a man can take a pill to get an erection doesn't mean he shouldn't look for the cause of his impotence and treat the etiology (doctor-speak for "reason for a medical problem"). What most men want and need is a complete

What most men want and need is a complete resolution of *all* symptoms from the hormone that made them virile and young for their first forty years: testosterone.

resolution of *all* symptoms from the hormone that made them virile and young for their first forty years: testosterone.

The following story is a tragic example of what can occur when doctors follow a thirty-year-old script they learned in medical school and don't keep up with modern research or the changes in medical thinking. Richard, a fifty-seven-year-old patient, has a story that breaks my heart.

When Richard came to see me for testosterone replacement, we determined that he was a prime candidate, and I put him on testosterone pellet therapy. Over the course of three years, he lost excess weight, managed to discontinue his medications (prescribed by his regular internal medicine doctor), and lowered his blood pressure to normal. A success by all accounts, Richard was happy, and I was proud of what we had achieved.

At that time, he went in for his annual checkup with his internist. The doctor raved about his own success as a physician and the progress he'd made to lower Richard's blood pressure and to help him lose weight and decrease his BMI. Richard, now sixty, was a prime example of the benefits of testosterone replacement therapy, but the doctor was unaware that his key to health was testosterone pellets.

Shocked by his doctor's arrogant attitude, Richard told him he believed the testosterone pellets were the direct cause of his health improvements. The doctor was outraged, and he shamed Richard. He told him in no uncertain terms that testosterone replacement therapy—which he'd been on for three years—would kill him, despite the progress he'd made. Because this therapy is not yet accepted standard medical practice, and even though Richard literally turned sickness back to health by using testosterone pellets, the doctor refused to look at the facts. He even predicted an early death for Richard! Richard was frightened and angry, and he knew the only thing that had improved his health over the past three years was testosterone pellets. So he fired the doctor and continued the pellets.

If you have a doctor like Richard's, you should consider doing exactly what Richard did. By the way, Richard is *still* healthy and vibrant—and he's *still* on testosterone.

Find Out If You Have TDS

The rest of this chapter allows you to self-assess whether you have TDS because the symptoms are listed and described. Simply check off the symptoms you have as you read the descriptions. The more symptoms you check off, the more likely it is that you have TDS.

You'll notice that the first six symptoms are all about sex. That's because men are most likely to recognize these symptoms of TDS first:

Six Symptoms of TDS:

- erectile dysfunction
- infrequent or decreased volume of ejaculation
- loss of sexual desire
- inability to achieve orgasm
- premature ejaculation
- loss of morning erections

By their mid-forties, men begin to feel a general loss of sex drive (libido). The time spent thinking about sex, talking about sex, planning sexual trysts, or watching porn decreases to once every few days or less. Sometimes this decreased obsession is a relief, but for most men it's a slow and insidious loss of what they've always known: a profound desire to initiate and seek out sexual activity.

And it's usually a surprise to them! They don't think of themselves as being old, and they don't expect this change. Of course, they know that some old men have trouble in *that* area, but they don't think it will happen to them when they're only forty, fifty, or even sixty! They always feel they're too young to lose interest in sex, and I agree with them—no matter what their age!

If these six symptoms are familiar to you, then use the following symptom discussions to help you determine the severity of your problem. We'll help you figure out what to do if your symptoms indicate TDS.

❏ Erectile Dysfunction

"My erections have become more difficult to get and maintain. Sometimes I just can't get up for the game, or my erection goes away right after I get it. That's actually worse."

The Murpheys were in my office for their initial interview. My patient was Alec, and Mrs. Murphey sat a little behind him. He'd brought his wife along to make sure that he gave me the proper information. He knew he "checked out" when asked probing questions about his medical health or illnesses. What followed would have been funny if it wasn't so serious.

When I asked Alec if his erections were satisfactory, he said, "Of course!" But his wife, out of his field of vision, firmly swung her head from side to side saying silently, "No way!" He answered all the questions about sex as though he had no issues, but his wife gave me a negative headshake for each of his answers. I finally asked Mrs. Murphey to honestly tell us her opinion about their sex life.

She kindly patted him on the hand and said, "Honey, it just isn't the same anymore. In fact, you aren't really getting hard enough for us to have sex. I think you may be in denial."

Then Alec dropped the mask and admitted that the more he tried, the worse things got. He did need help. Testosterone pellets did the trick and his ED, as well as the other symptoms of TDS, were gone within a month. He came back by himself for his four-month follow-up visit and proudly told me that he was back to his youthful sexuality.

Although erections are primarily a function of blood flow, blood flow is secondary to an adequate testosterone level plus enough nitric oxide, the substance that Viagra® stimulates. Nitric oxide allows the blood vessels to dilate so the blood can flow into the penis.

All these factors must be addressed at the same office visit when testosterone pellets are inserted. Your doctor must review all signs and symptoms of disease or conditions that can impair a robust erection. The following list shows the necessary factors involved in having a normal, functional, and satisfying erection.

Good Erections Require:

- Adequate free testosterone blood level (>129 ng/ml)
- Adequate nitric oxide
- Good arterial blood flow without narrowed arteries secondary to plaque deposits or stimulants
- Sufficiently high blood pressure in the pelvis for an erection
- Normal blood glucose for good vascular dilation
- Normal nervous supply (no multiple sclerosis or other neurologic disease)

To make sure blood flow is adequate after you start testosterone therapy, it's imperative to fix the other factors that can be fixed while we're increasing your testosterone. It does you *no good* to treat only one factor that causes ED if there are other unresolved problems, because your erections won't be good enough to make you really hard. In fact, many studies indicate that men who ask for and receive only ED drugs to solve their sexual problems stop using them after a few months because the problem is *not* just a blood flow problem. The problem is a lack of desire, and they need T for that! Other factors, such as libido and emotional arousal, must be addressed, and these simply do not occur if your testosterone levels fall below total T of 400 ng/dl and free T of 129 ng/ml.

Doctors should evaluate your risks for arteriosclerosis (hardening of the arteries with lipid levels), take a history of heart attack or stroke, and test for early adult-onset diabetes (type 2), because these all affect erections. All of these problems, if present, must be treated for a man to have normal erections. In men who are over age fifty-five, there might be high blood pressure or arteries that either are stiff and no longer dilate or that are narrowed with plaque deposits that prevent blood flow to the penis. It's very important to determine a man's vascular health to make a reasonable prognosis about the effect of testosterone on ED.

Albert, a seventy-year-old man who had been a chronic smoker for fifty-five years, had recently suffered a heart attack. He came to me for testosterone replacement therapy because he thought that this would bring back his erections and help him regain his lost sex life. He didn't, however, tell me about his smoking history or his heart attack. When his pellet therapy failed to produce the results he expected, he was very angry with me for taking his money under "false pretenses."

When he brought his wife in with him to complain about the failed "promise" of testosterone replacement, I told them that he needed to see a vascular surgeon to evaluate the blood vessels in his pelvis. I recommended this because he had reported no history of vascular disease. At this point, his wife interrupted.

"Did he tell you he had a heart attack a year ago and was a chronic smoker for over fifty years? The man sleeps with oxygen!"

Albert became visibly angry with his wife. He had deliberately withheld that information in our initial interview because he was afraid I wouldn't proceed with the pellet therapy. What he didn't know was that there were other reasons I would have recommended pellet therapy—such as his osteoporosis and his general muscular weakness. But had I known about his vascular problems, I would also have told him that it was too late for the pellets to be a panacea for his erectile issues. Now I had to tell him that the only way for him to get the kind of erections he wanted was with a penile implant or some other device to help him get erect. The pellets wouldn't accomplish that because of his previous lifestyle choices and current vascular damage.

Most men aren't beyond our ability to help them regain satisfying erections, although I sometimes can't predict how testosterone replacement will influence their erections due to other medicines they take for chronic illnesses they may have (such as COPD) that testosterone can't overcome.

We frequently combine testosterone with supplements like L-arginine and Neo40® (over-the-counter supplements that increase nitric oxide and dilate pelvic blood vessels to achieve and optimize treatment for ED). We also add Viagra® or Cialis® to enhance the erections improved by testosterone pellet therapy if the other problems still impact the erection. Together, testosterone pellets and Viagra® or similar drugs work well to restore normal sexual function.

Further, taking testosterone helps you clean out the narrowed vessels from the plaques that decrease blood flow to the penis.

ED is not caused by low testosterone alone. It can be caused by other medical conditions and diseases, illegal substances, and medications. The following conditions and diseases can cause ED.

Causes of ED:

- High blood pressure
- Low blood pressure
- Heart failure
- Diabetes
- Chronic obstructive pulmonary disease (COPD)
- Coronary artery disease (atherosclerosis)
- Autoimmune disease
- Multiple sclerosis (MS)
- Surgical damage to the pudendal nerve branch of the internal iliac nerves
- Nerve compression in the lower back

These medications and illegal substances can make ED worse:

- Beta blockers (blood pressure medication)
- Diuretics ("water pills")
- High blood pressure medications
- Diet pills, amphetamines, medication for attention deficit disorder (ADD), cocaine
- Antipsychotic medications that increase prolactin
- Marijuana
- Opiates
- Antidepressants

Once we bring the testosterone level back to a young, normal male blood level (400-1,500 ng/dl), the presence of this hormone can decrease the effects of the other conditions and diseases shown on the previous page. Changing some types of drugs listed above to a different category of drug or a lower dose can also improve erectile function when combined with testosterone pellets.

Sometimes COPD—usually caused by years of smoking—can damage the lungs so badly that it causes hypoxia (low oxygen). This is what happened to Albert. Hypoxia makes the arteries constrict rather than dilate, which prevents a satisfying and functional erection. Some men's lungs and arteries are so severely damaged, like Albert's, that no amount of testosterone can overcome this effect. In those cases, we advocate oxygen therapy at night and Neo40®, a nitric oxide supplement that dilates blood vessels, and we try to replace or discontinue unnecessary medications that impair erectile function. while adding testosterone pellets to increase the blood level of testosterone. We may also refer the patient for penile implant surgery.

After we address the vascular problems that lead to erectile issues, we focus on other causes of ED beyond low testosterone.

A man can have ED and still have adequate levels of testosterone. For instance, type 2 diabetes, obesity, MS, and Muscular Dystrophy (MD) can also lead to ED. Doctors must know if a patient is suffering from any of these diseases to predict whether adding testosterone will help eliminate ED issues.

❏ Infrequent or Decreased Volume of Ejaculation

"I can't believe I'm telling you this, but it bothers me that I can't feel anything come out when I climax. It's really weird and doesn't seem normal!"

Jerry, a forty-five-year-old master carpenter, reluctantly told me this at his first office visit. Guys discuss this subject only when they're really bothered by it.

The production of semen is not necessary for satisfying sex; and most men say that if they had to choose one over the other, they'd pick orgasm over ejaculation. However, producing semen is a sign of being "normal," so most of my patients want to take the necessary steps to get back to normal, which includes testosterone pellets and doing whatever they can to produce semen. They're glad to know that a large volume of semen isn't necessary for satisfaction or for orgasm, but they want the same sensations they've always had.

Testosterone increases the production of semen from the prostate and seminal vesicles, but as testosterone decreases and nitric oxide is no longer plentiful in the blood vessels, ejaculatory volume becomes less and less over time. Yet there are other factors that can decrease the volume of ejaculate other than low T. These include dehydration, lack of amino acids arginine and ornithine, low DHT (dihydrotestosterone) and inadequate oxytocin (a hormone from the brain that is stimulated by free testosterone), various medications, elevated prolactin, and/or estrogen. All these can cause reduced volume of ejaculation.

The first step in recovering a normal ejaculate is to replace testosterone with pellets to bring the testosterone to a high enough level to stimulate the production of oxytocin and nitric oxide.

We often add supplements called arginine/ornithine and Neo40® to improve the volume by increasing the necessary amino acids and to increase vascular dilation that stimulate nitric oxide levels. The amount of ejaculate rarely returns to the normal volume that men had when they were in their twenties, but we can usually create a sufficient volume to satisfy most of our patients.

❏ Loss of Sexual Desire

"I really couldn't care less if I ever have sex again," Steve confessed. *"My wife came to see you and now she's ready to go. We've switched roles! I used to complain all the time that she wasn't interested and didn't initiate sex often enough, but now she's always after me to have sex. What's wrong with me? I'd rather take a nap, mow the lawn—anything but sex!"*

The strength of your sexual desire is determined by two factors: the need for sex and having a suitable partner. Many of my male patients remind me that their favorite partner is themselves because of their longstanding relationship with their own sex organs. But after that, a relationship is integral to feeling desire.

I've learned so much by treating thousands of men and women with testosterone, and I can tell you that sexual desire is purely chemical. The higher the blood level of testosterone, the more desire an individual will feel.

Some of us were born with higher blood levels of testosterone; others have high or low sensitivity to testosterone, but the blood level that can make or break a sex drive is variable between men. Without testosterone, most men would rather lay on the couch eating chips and watching football!

Michael is a very successful businessman who builds and sells companies. He came to me for testosterone at the request of a girlfriend—not his sexual partner—when he was forty. He confided that he had no sexual desire, and sex was literally off his radar. He claimed that he'd never had much desire, even when he was an adolescent.

I asked Michael when he'd reached puberty and about his growth spurt and his "hairiness." He said that he'd gotten tall but was always so overweight that he had trouble walking. He even had his man boobs surgically removed when he was in his twenties. It left his body scarred and unusual looking, and he regretted the surgery. (I always recommend meds to shrink man boobs rather than surgery because the surgery is always unsightly.)

Michael and I made a deal. I would oversee his medical, nutritional, and exercise regimens to see if we could get him to a place he'd never been—an environment with enough testosterone for him to have a good sex drive, where he could make muscle and lose weight so he could lose his now-regrown man boobs. He agreed to maintain an exercise program with a low-carb diet and very low intake of alcohol (which is hard to do in the business world).

Five months later, I didn't recognize him. Michael now lived half a country away, but he'd kept his word and lost almost one hundred pounds by having testosterone pellets inserted; taking Arimidex® (anastrozole), a drug to decrease his estrogen; incorporating proper supplements to keep his nutrition healthy, and exercising daily.

He told me that he now knew how other men felt. Before, he'd never had a hint of sexual desire, or felt manly, or had the joy of feeling his own muscles ripple—and now he felt all that and *had morning erections. Michael was on his way to being "normal" for the first time in his life!*

All the doctors that money could buy hadn't discovered the basic problem that caused Michael's trouble: a lack of testosterone and the conversion of testosterone to estrogen in the fat.

Michael is a new man, and the last time I saw him, another gorgeous patient in my office hit on him and asked him out to dinner.

Many patients who've never been able to have an adequate erection or who've never felt the fun of the sexual dance are simply deficient in one thing: testosterone. These men and women have never experienced orgasms or had the desire to have one; but when they come to my office, after four to five months of treatment, the fire has been lit. They tell me in various words, "Now I know what everyone's been talking about!" And they give a smile that shows their satisfaction with being "normal"!

If the amount of testosterone in the blood is the key, then is it the *total* testosterone level (active and inactive) or the *free T* (the amount of active testosterone) that makes the difference? In my vast experience, the total T level has nothing to do with how men feel or if they can have an erection. But having a *free T* level above 129 ng/ml is key for a man to have normal function.

Of course, desire begins in the brain. When the "free" form of testosterone crosses the blood-brain barrier, it causes men (and women) to think about sex, fantasize about it, plan for it, and look for opportunities to have it, as well as initiate sex with their partner. Without free T, there's no desire and sex becomes a burden—or even work! It may be enjoyable once it starts, but the desire to have sex is missing.

Men who have always had a great sexual appetite—and a generous amount of free T—find the lack of desire disturbing. They aren't themselves anymore, and this symptom of low T is devastating to their ego. They question themselves and their relationships instead of checking their hormones.

This particular symptom of TDS breaks up the fabric of family life, and their children—as well as their mates—are left wondering what hit them.

In the end, lack of desire has a lot to do with male andropause, the time when some men chase new cars, status, and maybe another partner in order to prove themselves. This particular symptom of TDS breaks up the fabric of family life, and their children—as well as their mates—are left wondering what hit them. Replacing testosterone and achieving a youthful level of free T is key to regenerating sexual desire.

As men get older, they often make more and more estrogen, which binds the testosterone so that it can't cross the blood-brain barrier to stimulate the brain. In such cases, we use a supplement called DIM (diindolylmethane) and a drug called Arimidex® in our testosterone pellets to block the production of estrone and estradiol—the causes of low free T. Arimidex® and DIM raise the free T percentage to a normal level, so there's enough active T to get to the brain and create desire.

Antidepressants can also cause a loss of desire. Many people who take antidepressants find that their desire to have sex has disappeared. They also find that even if they're stimulated by their partner, they often suddenly lose interest or are unable to finish with an orgasm. This can leave a man and his partner in a state of confusion and hurt. Who did something wrong? Who is no longer attractive? Who has fallen out of love? The answer is *none of the above.* The problem is chemical. Talk to your doctor about your options to improve your sexual desire when taking an antidepressant.

❑ Inability to Achieve an Orgasm

When Jack sat at the consultation table in my office, he looked like a big bear ready to strike. I'd never met him before, but I had his labs and medical history committed to memory. He was a serious guy and was quite disturbed about something. I guessed that it was because he didn't want to be there or one of his symptoms was completely stressing him.

He addressed me as "Hey, Doc," and told me that he'd been in the military in his early years.

"This whole getting older thing is killing me! I don't have a need to have sex, but my wife thinks something's fishy. So to prove to her that I love her, I spend all day revving myself up for sex when I get home. Then I break out the Viagra®, and all the plumbing is working just fine. But when we're almost "there," I can't finish! It takes minutes, then an hour. By then we've both lost interest and I just quit! I'm frustrated and mad at my damn body! It doesn't work anymore! You've got to fix me!"

Climax, or orgasm, is the emotional and physical release after a sexual encounter. The swelling and other physical changes that are characteristic of the stage of sex prior to orgasm do not subside unless climax is reached, which makes the inability to climax uncomfortable and frustrating. A lack of testosterone may cause a lack of orgasm. It also causes an inability to get an erection and to ejaculate, but these symptoms usually present in a cluster rather than one at a time. They rarely exist when there is plenty of free T in the blood. Low free T in the blood stream, by contrast, will cause an inability to climax, to ejaculate, and to have an erection.

Frustration is the primary result for both men and women who can't receive the endorphin benefit of sex. More women than men can't achieve orgasm, which makes it that much harder on men who have this problem.

Frustration is the primary result for both men and women who can't receive the endorphin benefit of sex that culminates in an orgasm.

It's generally a testosterone production problem; however, sometimes other drugs can interfere with orgasm—and no one warns you about this! If a man can't achieve orgasm after we treat him with testosterone pellets and everything else is working well, we look for medications and supplements that block orgasm.

The list is short, but many men take these drugs.

<u>Drugs That Can Impair Orgasm:</u>

- Antidepressants
- Antipsychotics
- Mood stabilizers
- Proscar® (finasteride)
- Propecia® (finasteride)
- Duteraside
- Diet pills

- Medications for attention deficit disorder (ADD) and attention deficit hyperactivity disorder (ADHD) and other amphetamines
- Beta blockers

If the problem still persists after we've achieved an excellent level of free T, we ask the primary care doctor or other physician who treats the our patients to change their choice of drug to something less deleterious to orgasm. Usually, after a switch from an antidepressant like Prozac®, Celexa®, Lexapro®, or Zoloft® to Wellbutrin® everything resolves. Even better news is that most of the time, men who take T pellets and are on antidepressants find that after their T level returns to normal, they don't need antidepressants anymore.

> Most of the time, men who take T pellets and are on antidepressants find that after their T level returns to normal, they don't need antidepressants anymore.

❏ Premature Ejaculation

Once in a while, we treat guys who can get an erection but are so stimulated that they ejaculate prematurely. They can't sustain their erection without coming quickly, which is, of course, disappointing for their partner. In these cases, the same antidepressants that *prevent ejaculation* in some men work well to *prolong erections* in others, so they can enjoy sex for more than a minute or two.

❏ Loss of Morning Erections

"Do you have a male doctor here that I can talk to? I don't think you'll understand this particular problem," Hunter said to me as he contemplated his shoelaces.

I leaned back and told him that after thirty-nine years in medicine, I'd heard it all. *"Talk to me like I'm a friend or a nurse,"* I said. After considering this approach, he haltingly began his story.

> *"Since I was eleven or even younger I had a hard-on every morning. It got to be like an old friend that woke me up. It made me feel alive. But now I'm forty-five and it's gone! I feel old and out of sync. What can I do? Will testosterone make it come back?"*

I confess, I didn't realize the importance of this "secret male sign" that most men find reassuring. I wasn't taught to ask about morning erections in my training, and it wasn't on the intake questionnaire as one of the signs that a man's testosterone was low. But after just a few months of taking care of men and their hormones, the crucial nature of this physical expression that signifies youth became obvious, and I started to ask about it in my office consultations. The lack of morning erections seems to be a very important predictor of erectile function, as it's unconscious and is rarely affected by the psychological factors that may affect erectile function.

After I placed my male patients on testosterone pellets, I learned to ask them if they were getting morning erections. If a man said that he had morning erections but couldn't be erect for sex, the problem was not physical. ED that continues after normal Free T levels are achieved and morning erections return is usually caused by emotional and relational issues, rather than by the physical ability to have and maintain an erection.

It helps to talk to men about what sex therapists would refer to as *stage fright*. This is when a man develops performance anxiety because of his fear of failure in regard to his erection and his ability to satisfy his partner. Stage fright can happen for many reasons, not including the lack of testosterone. So if a man has a normal free T level, we must look into other potential causes and perhaps make a referral for counseling for the couple (see more in chapter 5).

If you want to evaluate yourself for ED, which generally means low T, consider if you are still greeted each morning with an erection. If you have morning erections, then perhaps your ED is situational, not hormonal.

Marcus and Lilly came to see me together because after forty-five years of marriage, they no longer wanted to have sex. During our interview together, Lilly cast a lot of the blame on Marcus. She belittled him at every turn. He just took it and slid down farther in his chair until he was in a slump.

"Of course I can't get excited about sex," she said. "You're limp, and it just lets me down when we try to be intimate!"

At that point, I asked Lilly to step out of the room so I could interview Marcus alone.

"Is this a typical conversation between you and your wife?" I asked.

Marcus looked at the floor and said, "Yes."

"I can fix your body," I said, "so that you can have physical intimacy, but it won't solve the problem. Part of the problem is that your relationship's been damaged—probably due to your ED in the beginning—and now your wife has gotten angry. Let's work on the physical side, and I'll refer you to Brett Newcomb to heal the wounds in your relationship."

I treated Marcus with both T and Viagra® for his ED. It took a little more than a year for him and his wife to reestablish their trust so that they could have a satisfying, intimate relationship. They rediscovered their love and affection for one another, and their sex life improved dramatically.

❑ Loss of Muscle Mass

"Where are my muscles? I've lost strength and stamina, and my muscular body has developed into a beer belly! This has to be a bad dream!"

Tim, at fifty-five, came to me with the complaint that his body didn't respond to his diet and workout regimen anymore. Even though he did resistance training with heavy weights, his arms were still soft and flabby, his belly was was large and soft, and his six-pack was a thing of the past. He felt that his change in diet and the intensity of his workouts should have made a difference. But all he got from working out was tired. He did not get a better body.

> *What Tim didn't know was that he didn't have enough testosterone to grow the muscle mass he was seeking. Testosterone is essential for building both bone and muscle. A man who's over age fifty will not get the results he seeks by simply working out and changing his eating habits. He needs to raise his testosterone to the level he had in earlier years.*

It doesn't matter what symptom brings a man to my office; by the end of the appointment, we usually get around to the pain he feels about losing his strength, skeletal muscle mass, and youthful body shape. It's somewhat embarrassing for them to talk about, even though it's quite important. Men hate to seem vain, so talking with me about their body image is often uncomfortable. For men, a youthful body means having defined muscles in the upper body, lack of belly fat, and a full head of hair. They miss these physical signs of youth when they're gone, and they can't get them back without testosterone. What they don't realize is that their bodily appearance can actually be a sign of a real medical problem, not just an accident of nature or a failure of will and masculinity.

Testosterone is the hormone that controls the qualities that make men attractive to themselves and to females, and in some cases other male admirers. Believe it or not, there's a competition for men to look younger than their same-aged friends. Men are very competitive, so don't let them tell you they don't care about how they look. They do! They may not know what to do to fix it, but I do!

I call treating men with testosterone pellets a *two-fer*. It's a two-for-one solution because the added testosterone stimulates the pituitary gland to produce human growth hormone (HGH).

The only form of testosterone that brings men back to a youthful, muscled body is T pellets, which stimulate GH better than all other forms of T replacement. My patients don't usually require growth hormone supplementation in addition to T pellets until they're quite advanced in years—over seventy-five. The fact that they can receive both testosterone *and* an increase in GH for the price of just T pellets makes the pellets the most cost-effective treatment of choice. Together, these hormones cause overall fat loss, belly fat loss, increased lean body mass, increased energy, growth of hair and nails, and a faster metabolism, which results in what we recognize as male beauty!

Taking high-priced HGH injections costs between $1,200 and $1,700 per month. The cost of male T pellets averages only $225 per month, and you get the benefit of both when taking T pellets without the high cost of HGH.

John came to see me primarily because he was a weight lifter and a self-proclaimed exercise nut. When he turned fifty-eight, it all went to pieces. He claimed that the more hours he worked out, the more muscle he lost. Worse yet, he no longer got the runner's high after exercising; he just got severely fatigued and needed a nap. The one pleasurable thing he'd had to relieve stress had disappeared in his middle fifties, and he was miserable! With nothing left to try, he began medicating his anxiety and depression with alcohol and cookies. By the time he got to my office, he was fifty pounds overweight, depressed, and fatigued. He was so desperate to get back to normal that he would've have done anything I suggested to get better. And he did.

John was one of my favorite patients because he followed the playbook exactly as I advised. He got T pellets, immediately cut out alcohol, and went on the diet I recommend to my male patients (see appendix C), Dr. Maupin's Low-Carb Diet. He also took his supplements of DIM (diindolylmethane) for belly fat, pregnenalone for DHEA and DHT production, methylated B vitamins, arginine ornithine (building blocks for muscle), and endodren, an animal adrenal pill that suppresses the cortisol surges that accompany anxiety attacks.

John is an engineer. He made graphs of his exercise program, weight, and water intake. He impressed me with his dedication, and his outcome was no less miraculous. In four months, he lost fifty pounds—most of that was fat—and he gained ten pounds of muscle! He conquered the problems caused by lost testosterone and his own self-medication. He'd found the correct treatment, and he was sticking with it!

John resolved all of his symptoms of aging with T pellets and supplements, but the most important result to him was that his exercise decreased his stress again and made his body beautiful too.

I could write an entire book about the unbelievable outcomes I've seen in my male patients because of T pellets. But it is the *how* as much as the *what* that you need to know, so you can decide whether to receive T pellet treatment and then learn *how* to make it work to reach your goals.

You may not understand the physiology of muscles, but the building blocks of muscle come primarily from red meat. It's difficult to make muscle if you don't eat enough red meat. Combining proper diet with the ideal workout is necessary to get your strength and muscle mass back. The ideal workout includes using weights every other day. Muscle breaks down when you exercise, and it builds back up the day after your workout. You must rest the part of your body you worked the day after resistance exercise to truly build up muscle.

The day of your workout, your body breaks down the building blocks of muscle and excretes them. The following day, you create new muscle where the old muscle used to be, and you build more than the amount of muscle you had to begin with. If you don't eat too many carbs, you'll use the fat that runs through your muscles (like in a ribeye steak) for energy, and your muscle becomes more compact and defined. When you work out again, the process starts over.

How muscles are built on the microscopic level is complex, but I'll try to explain. Testosterone stimulates the growth of muscle and stimulates human growth hormone (HGH). HGH then stimulates the construction of larger and larger *myotubules*, which make very strong muscles. Think of many cylindrical tubes that support a building with greater strength than a series of 2x4s or dowels. A man literally gets a stronger and sturdier body constructed of stronger muscles when he replaces his lost testosterone with T pellets.

When we age without T, loss of muscle mass can cause severe problems. When it's severe and is evident throughout the body, it causes weakness and frailty and impairs a man's ability to live independently. We call that *sarcopenia*. This condition is secondary to testosterone loss in the extreme and results in a man looking old, wasted, and frail. You'll read more about this condition in chapter 3 where the diseases caused by long-term testosterone deficiency are discussed.

❑ Loss of Stamina and Strength

"I've always been an athlete," Dave emphasized, "and I used to look great; but you wouldn't know it now. I can't get through a full workout. I get out of breath and I'm weak. I've had to shorten the same workouts I've been doing since I played football in college! And when I'm finished at the gym, instead of feeling energized and ready for anything, I feel like I need a nap and I can't go on. The worst part is that I ache in every area that I worked out. My muscles ache so much that I can't move. I've tried magnesium and water, electrolytes, and eating before, during, and after exercising. What's wrong with me?"

Dave was very distraught that his life had changed so dramatically. I've heard this complaint so many times that I could confidently tell him that testosterone pellets would bring him back to normal within a few months. I know the need for athletes to exercise regularly and to push themselves to the limit in order for them to feel well and healthy. Testosterone is the single necessary substance to reverse weak muscles.

Dave had poor stamina because without T, the muscles don't get enough blood flow to support long exercise sessions. The restricted blood flow means that his muscles were screaming for oxygen, which leaves the muscle with a garbage problem: the lactic acid that builds up and is normally swept away with good blood flow just sits in the muscle because of a lack of blood flow. Lactic acid can cause the muscles to ache and cramp for days after only one exercise session. Without T, exercise becomes unbearable!

Dave's final complaint was that he no longer got the "feel good" feeling—he just felt tired. Testosterone supplies the good endorphins and norepinephrine in the brain that give runners the runner's high. Exercise carries free T into the brain to stimulate endorphins and other neurotransmitters.

❑ Poor Recovery After a Heart Attack

The heart muscle is made of specialized striated muscle and is like the skeletal muscles in your body, except it has a slightly different structure. When the heart is damaged from lack of oxygen from a clogged artery (a heart attack), the muscle that was previously part of the heart—that did the work of pumping blood—dies. Rather than leaving a hole in your heart, it creates a scar that doesn't stretch like the muscle once did. The dead muscle doesn't grow back. Normally, a person is left with a scarred heart that isn't as strong as it was before. Not only does this scarred heart not push out as much blood volume to the body, it now pushes with less force.

Drew had a heart attack shortly after starting pellets. Both his cardiologist and I agreed that this event had been building for at least a decade prior to the event and that the testosterone was not the cause. Drew recovered very quickly from the heart attack that destroyed one-quarter of his heart muscle, and he asked his cardiologist if he could stay on testosterone pellets. He'd felt so good on them, but they were beginning to wear off as he was completing his cardiotherapy. His cardiologist asked me for literature about how testosterone strengthens the heart and improves recovery after a heart attack; after reading the material, he agreed that Drew should remain on the pellets.

What came next was a surprise to this experienced cardiologist and to me. Drew's heart muscle did not scar, and his heart did not weaken! Instead, his heart was stronger than it was before the heart attack, and he had no residual shortness of breath or trouble exercising aerobically for more than an hour! Of course, the heart attack frightened him, so he lost sixty pounds and stopped drinking. He'd had a scare, but he had no lasting damage to his heart.

Drew is grateful to God for this warning sign and for his full recovery. He and his cardiologist attributed his amazing recovery to his dieting, exercising, and testosterone pellets.

These findings are supported by many studies, primarily in European medical studies. For some reason, American doctors don't usually hear about testosterone pellets helping a patient recover from the damage caused by a heart attack.

❏ Insomnia / Poor Quality Sleep

Insomnia is defined as trouble getting to sleep or staying asleep, or sleep that doesn't result in feeling rested. Men who experience insomnia from low T fall asleep easily, but they wake up in the early hours and can't go back to sleep. Some wake up and go to the bathroom every few hours, which is also related to low T. As a result, they feel exhausted all day.

Carl's primary reason for seeing me was his poor sleep. He'd already undergone a sleep study that proved normal, he'd had a neurology consultation and an EEG, and the treating physicians said he was fine. He knew he wasn't. I was the last stop on his search to find a good night's sleep.

"No matter what I try, I can't stay asleep!" Carl complained. He'd always been a deep sleeper and had taken his refreshing sleep for granted until he turned fifty.

"I'm constantly exhausted, and when I get up in the morning after waking up many times through the night, I'm as exhausted as when I went to bed! I sometimes wonder why I try to sleep at all. I've been given sleeping pills, which help me go to sleep, but I still wake up at 2:00 a.m. and can't go back to sleep until it's time to get up at 6:00 a.m. The sleeping pills leave me feeling hung over, and not only am I exhausted all the time, I'm all tied up with anxiety. If testosterone can help me with this, I'll be your spokesman!"

I've found that people who are sleepless from TDS—rather than from untreated ADHD, anxiety, elevated cortisol, worry, brain injury, and other neurologic conditions—experience the following.

Insomnia Caused by Low Testosterone:
- They never had insomnia before age forty.
- They can always fall asleep.
- They sleep for only short periods of time.
- They wake for no reason around 2 a.m. or 3 a.m. and can't get back to sleep.
- They don't dream.
- Their sleep tests are usually normal.
- They often have restless legs.
- They always wake up as tired as when they went to bed.
- The lack of sleep plus TDS causes weight gain, which leads to snoring and can lead to an inaccurate medical diagnosis of sleep apnea.

These expressions of insomnia are quite different from other causes of insomnia. Trying testosterone pellets as a test is the best way to diagnose sleep issues caused by TDS. If insomnia is caused by low T, you should get better within six weeks of starting T pellets.

TDS insomnia is characterized by waking up tired and never feeling refreshed. A man who has enough testosterone will describe his sleep as deep, restful, healing sleep with rapid eye movement (REM) and dreaming. During REM sleep, we repair our cells, work out our psychological problems, and rest our brain, refreshing it for the day to come. Sounds amazing, doesn't it?

Without adequate testosterone, we go to sleep easily and progress through the first two stages of sleep. But when it comes time to enter stages three and four—REM sleep—we wake up. We never, or only briefly, enter the last two stages. This process recurs again and again throughout the night and leaves us exhausted and unable to feel fully awake during the day.

My testosterone-deprived male patients remind me of the plight of the Greek god Sisyphus. He was eternally doomed to push a heavy boulder up a mountain. When he finally reached the top, he watched the boulder slip away and roll back down the mountain. He was condemned to keep pushing this boulder up the mountain to see it slip away, only to push it up the mountain again.

Most of my patients say that going through the first two stages of sleep, only to wake up and go back to stage one again, creates that same feeling. Like Sisyphus, they are condemned to try to reach a goal, only to almost get there and start over again. Night after night, the process never ends. Without testosterone, this tortured sleep pattern is replicated in many men and women over the age of fifty who don't take testosterone. Sound familiar?

Even though insomnia results in fatigue, fatigue and insomnia are two different issues. A man may have fatigue as a result of insomnia, but he can also develop fatigue without insomnia. Insomnia leaves him too tired to enjoy life and leads to lowered immunity, higher risk of accidents, and lower productivity. Interestingly, insomnia is twice as prevalent among women than among men, which follows the gender difference in blood levels of testosterone. Men produce ten times the testosterone of women. On average, women also become testosterone deficient ten years before men, so their insomnia and fatigue begin earlier in their lives.

I'm amazed that we keep developing new sleep drugs that treat the symptom—insomnia—but don't offer true restful sleep by providing bioidentical testosterone replacement to both men and women. I blame the FDA and the medical-pharma conglomerate that ignores the role of testosterone to treat age-related insomnia.

"Testosterone replacement has made such a positive difference in my life. I no longer suffer from tension headaches, and I sleep through the night feeling rested," Carl exclaimed during our follow-up

Replacing the most important hormone that you had in your youth is the most normal thing you can do to improve your health.

consultation. It had been four months since his first testosterone pellet insertion. "My energy has dramatically increased, and I feel whole again! One hormone has now replaced three drugs that I used to take for sleep and tension headaches."

The long-term lack of sleep can change a man's personality and make him physically ill. It affects his relationships, sex drive, mood, and job performance—and it impairs his immune system, so he gets sick more often.

Men who refuse to try testosterone as a remedy for insomnia may not understand that insomnia leads to other symptoms and illnesses. If this is your attitude, consider this: replacing the most important hormone that you had in your youth is the most normal thing you can do to improve your health.

If you accept insomnia as your new norm and avoid testosterone replacement, you will in all likelihood watch your body and mind deteriorate as you experience more and more sickness and fatigue. It takes about ten years after your first symptoms of insomnia-related TDS before you begin to see your health deteriorate, so please consider the future and use the knowledge that medical researchers have given us to prevent future illness.

❑ Fatigue

Tom literally threw his body in the chair and slumped down. He was only forty-five but looked fifty-five. He had deep circles under his eyes, greyish skin, and an unfocused stare that reminded me of what I looked like after thirty-six hours on call as a resident in OB/GYN.

He took some deep breaths as if there wasn't enough oxygen in the room and told me, "I wake up every morning and wish I could crawl back in bed—every day! I am soooooo tired! I still go to work, but my performance is down and I'm worried about keeping my job.

"At night, I fall asleep right away; but no matter how many things

I try, I can't stay asleep through the night. I wake up at 2:55 a.m. and can't go back to sleep. I never dream. I'm so frustrated!

"But it's not just the sleep. I can't work in the yard all day like I used to. After only two hours, my arms and legs ache for the next two days. I need a nap in the afternoon and just stare at the computer. Is my life over at forty-five?"

Tom had acute and severe fatigue that T pellets would remedy, but he'd waited so long to get help that it would take four to six months to get complete relief. Fatigue is characterized by a lack of energy and low motivation to initiate any activity. Men who are fatigued feel like they drag themselves through their day.

Fatigue is one of the most common symptoms that patients complain about to their doctors. It's also one of most elusive symptoms to diagnose. It can result from a busy life, a virus, hormonal deficiency, low blood sugar, cancer, or a blood disorder as common as anemia or as dangerous as leukemia.

Because there are many potential causes of fatigue, it's important to have a full medical evaluation to rule out the most dangerous and most common causes. The most common causes of fatigue include the following.

Common Causes of Fatigue:
- Insomnia; sleep disorders leading to daytime fatigue
- Hypothyroidism (low thyroid)
- Stress and the hormonal imbalance that comes from it (high cortisol)
- Hypoglycemia (low blood sugar)
- Lack of exercise
- Anemia
- Depression
- Poor diet: lack of protein, vitamins, and overall nutrition

- Chronic fatigue caused by the mononucleosis virus
- Untreated attention deficit disorder (ADD) and attention deficit hyperactivity disorder (ADHD)
- Cardiac arrhythmia and heart failure
- Hypopituitary (low pituitary) hormones
- Medications (beta blockers, hypertensives, sedatives, and antidepressants)

When all of these problems have been ruled out, we are left to consider TDS as a source of fatigue.

Testosterone is a wonderful, stimulating hormone of youth and energy. After a life of having his brain and body bathed in testosterone, the lack of testosterone creates a completely different environment for a man. It's like going to sleep in your own bed and waking up in another country. Our patients usually don't prioritize fatigue as what bothers them most, but at their follow-up visit after their first dose of testosterone pellets, they always comment on how good they feel and how much they can do now with their new-found energy. One memorable guy named Scott could hardly believe the difference in his energy since his pellets were inserted.

"You can't imagine the difference in my life! I had whittled my life down to work, eating, and trying to sleep. I had cancelled my other activities and limited my interaction with friends just so I could lie down and ... not sleep! I felt weak and fat and out of balance. Then I got the pellets and three weeks later, my wife looked a lot cuter than she had in my fog. We had sex for the first time in two years. Then I started calling up my golf buddies that I'd been too tired to see before, and now I play golf every Saturday morning. The honey-do list is even getting shorter. It's a miracle!"

Scott had lost his energy and his life when his testosterone disappeared, and now he had it back. It was his miracle!

❏ Memory Problems

Our brain and spirit, as well as the ability to remember everything that's happened in our lives, is what makes us human. When our memory is threatened, we start to fade away as a member of human society. That's why it's so terrifying to lose your ability to recall people's names, the names of places, and specific descriptive words used in conversation. When this happens, we often fear that we might have developed Alzheimer's disease or another dementia.

There's a specific type of memory loss that's characteristic of TDS. It's the loss of the ability to "label" people, places, and things with an appropriate name. Without this capability, we feel uneducated, or old, or demented. Luckily, it's reversible if treatment with testosterone pellets takes place within ten years after a man's testosterone drops below young healthy levels.

Jerry, a forty-five-year-old NFL coach, sat down in my office just after the season ended. He sighed and looked blankly at the floor. His big shoulders sagged, and he looked so much smaller than his 6' 3" height. When I asked him why he'd come to see me and what his worst symptoms were, he barely spoke. He had to fish around for words like my eighty-year-old grandmother did. He was terrified—and I was as well. I wondered if he'd endured so many concussions that I wouldn't be able to bring him back to complete health. After all, he was only in his forties. He had small children and a lovely wife; he should have his whole life ahead of him.

I did most of the talking and wrote everything down for his wife to read, so he didn't have to remember what we talked about. I prescribed testosterone pellets and a few necessary supplements meant to optimize the effectiveness of the testosterone. I also ordered blood work for four months from that day, and he scheduled an appointment for five months later. Then I led him to the exam room for his pellets. He didn't seem to be all there. I hoped to meet his real self in a few months.

Jerry never called or emailed in the intervening months, so I wasn't hopeful for a complete recovery. I can't tell you how shocked I was when I saw him again. He stood to his full height, shook my hand, and said my name! He was literally a different man—confident, articulate, and well-spoken. I didn't recognize him at first, and when I realized who he was, I couldn't stop smiling all day.

I've never seen anything more dramatic with any treatment available in medicine for memory loss. Jerry had experienced over seven hundred concussions starting at age ten (according to him). He was a tight-end in college and in the NFL and got tackled by larger players every time he received the ball. Now he's coaching an NFL team and is out of harm's way. After all those years of overextending his body and enduring recurrent concussions, he now can perform his job as a coach and has healed his brain with testosterone. His recovery is proof that replacing testosterone with T pellets can change lives.

How does this work? We know that the hormone testosterone is anabolic and builds and repairs tissue in every organ system. As we grow old, our perfectly balanced system of growth and breakdown becomes imbalanced in favor of decomposition. We become *catabolic*, and our bodies break down more cells than we grow. Bones become thin, our brains shrink, muscles atrophy, and we feel, look, and act old.

The loss of testosterone and growth hormone initiates this imbalance. Growth and repair are controlled by GH and testosterone. The breakdown is controlled by a lack of these hormones and a prevalence of the hormone cortisol.

When we are young, testosterone and growth hormone are the primary hormones in the brain that stimulate cell growth to replace dead cells and neurons. As we get older, we hit a critically low level of testosterone, below which our brain begins to shrink. We lose neurons daily, and it becomes more and more difficult to think and communicate. Testosterone promotes blood flow to the memory areas of the brain; the lack of it diverts blood flow from those areas and deprives the recall areas of the brain of oxygen. Both deficient oxygen and further breakdown of cells cause our brains to shrink from testosterone deficiency. However, if we replace testosterone through pellets, we can *sustain* the size of our brain and *maintain* our ability to think and remember.

Other functions of testosterone in the brain prevent dementia and Alzheimer's disease. Testosterone sustains blood flow to the area that contains short-term labeling memory and 3-D spatial visualization. Without sufficient T, the blood flow is shunted away from that area and, over time, we lose those brain functions due to hypoxia (low oxygen from poor blood flow).

Testosterone also stimulates the production of neurotransmitters (brain communicators) such as norepinephrine, dopamine, endorphins, and serotonin. Without T, this production decreases and repair of the cells that produce those neurotransmitters is also reduced. The loss of these neurotransmitters affects mood, balance, sleep, energy, cognition, immune function, and behavior.

There are two other functions of testosterone, both metabolic: anti-inflammatory activity and insulin sensitivity. There are two beliefs about Alzheimer's disease that are of interest. The first says that the disease is caused by inflammation that forms plaques on the neurons in the brain and kills them. The second theory is that Alzheimer's disease should be called type 3 diabetes. Adult diabetes causes insulin insensitivity, which damages the neurons. The insulin-sensitizing property of testosterone decreases the risk of "type 3 diabetes" in the brain and, therefore, Alzheimer's disease. The effect, however, is protective only if testosterone is replaced within ten years of the first symptoms of testosterone loss (like ED), so don't wait.

❏ Joint Aches / Arthritis

"Every muscle in my body aches, and my joints feel like they are grinding with every movement." Dan, a software designer with four kids, sighed. "I used to work out every day, played sports, and played basketball with my office team until I was fifty. Now I'm fifty-five and I can't move! I've seen a whole slew of doctors from orthopedic

surgeons to rheumatologists, homeopaths, and chiropractors, and no one has helped me! I'm at my wit's end. I need help yesterday!"

Joint and muscle aches are a common complaint of men with TDS, and these symptoms are rarely treated successfully by anything other than testosterone replacement. Testosterone has the magical quality of decreasing inflammation throughout the body and "oiling" all the joints. It increases the production of synovial fluid and treats any joint that has not been irreversibly damaged by friction.

The plethora of joint replacements in the US is evidence of two things about modern Western society. First, we push sports to the limit and damage our joints. As we age, we don't moderate our level of trauma to our joints. Second, we exercise aggressively long after our testosterone levels have dropped. If we fail to replace our testosterone and continue to exercise, we cause irreversible damage. Joint replacement may be the only cure.

I suggest that men over fifty moderate their exercise if they're not going to replace their testosterone. However, my preference is that aging men who like to exercise replace their testosterone before they damage their joints and ligaments. Replacing your testosterone with pellets will help you avoid the need for most joint replacements.

Dan, the software designer mentioned earlier, experienced excellent results. His joints began to feel better within four months of receiving T pellets, and by six months, all his joint pain was a distant memory.

❏ Poor Balance / Coordination

At forty-nine, Jim had had an active life. But he'd begun to notice that his balance was off. His golf game crashed, and he'd fallen down several times in the last year when he was running half marathons. This had never happened to him before. He also used to be a big hitter on his men's softball team, but now his timing was off. He was afraid he had a progressive illness like MS, or ALS, or some other neuromuscular disease that would eventually take his life. He could barely whisper these fears to me.

Jim's imbalance and poor coordination weren't from a progressive neuromuscular disease. They were from a loss of testosterone, which had affected his brain and inner ear—as well as his muscle strength. It had impaired his ability to balance with the trunk muscles of his back and abdomen.

Poor balance isn't usually the presenting (or most important) symptom my patients have, but when they have it, it causes them to avoid many activities they enjoyed when they were younger. I'm amazed at the number of men whose balance is key in their jobs as well as their after-work entertainment. Linemen, contractors, painters—even surgeons—need good balance to get through their day.

Testosterone reestablishes the neurologic pathways in the brain that are necessary for balance. It also directs blood to the area of the brain that controls musculoskeletal balance. That's the work testosterone does *centrally* (in the brain). But it also builds abdominal and back muscles that have become weak, despite exercise and weight lifting. The mass of muscles around the trunk of the body stabilizes us and gives us the ability to balance on one leg, walk the line, or climb a ladder to the roof and get back down.

Long-term balance problems caused by TDS can turn you into an old man in a nursing home who can't balance enough to stand or walk without assistance or a walker. That's what we want to avoid. Testosterone supports muscle and nerve regeneration without end, as long as it's continually replaced.

Four months after getting testosterone pellets, Jim returned to golf and softball. He had a renewed confidence and his golf score was better than ever. He didn't rely on his balance and coordination in his work, but being able to do the things that make life worthwhile is often just as important to a man as putting food on the table.

❏ The All-American Beer Belly

Go to the ballpark in any city on a Sunday afternoon, and you'll see a few thousand men with bulging beer bellies. Abdominal obesity is rampant in America. To me, this is the most obvious sign of the pervasiveness of TDS. If these guys sat around with their shirts off, they'd look like they were nine months pregnant. I think of how high their estrogen levels are and how low their free testosterone levels must be. They all need a diet, less alcohol, testosterone pellets, and a lot of exercise.

They often have a matching accessory: man boobs. The lower the level of free testosterone, together with the higher level of estrogen, causes both breast development and belly fat accumulation in men. The increased estrogen makes more fat, and the cycle continues from low T to high estrogen to more breast tissue and belly fat, which then again makes more estrogen and less T.

Testosterone pellets are not always enough to interrupt this awful cycle, so we either add Arimidex® to the pellets to lower estrogens or have men take it orally. That's the best combination to decrease breast tissue and belly fat in men.

Belly fat is the worst fat that we make. Not only is it unattractive to view, it also increases cholesterol, triglycerides, and cortisol. All of these lipid and hormone changes are triggered by low testosterone, and they can lead to heart attack, stroke, diabetes, impotence, and death.

These diseases are usually irreversible, and they consume all your time and assets in the struggle to stay alive.

Before you decide to ignore your beer belly because it's so easy to do nothing, consider how hard it will be to treat the diseases that can follow: diabetes, heart disease, osteoporosis, and dementia. These diseases are usually irreversible, and they consume all your time and assets in the struggle to stay alive. In the long run, it's truly easier to diet, exercise, and take testosterone pellets now.

By itself, a beer belly won't kill you, but it's a sign of medical problems that can—and will. The solution is simple: insert testosterone pellets twice a year and follow a low-carb diet, exercise regularly, and apply a little self-discipline. This is the recipe for keeping you healthy so you can enjoy a long, productive life.

❑ Ringing in the Ears

Barry is a very young sixty-five. He had many symptoms of TDS that were remedied by his first dose of pellets; his favorite benefit was that testosterone cured his ringing in the ears (tinnitus). He told me that tinnitus was like a chronic itch or like listening to dissonant music, but now what he heard was a sweet silence. Within four months, he seemed less anxious, and he stopped gritting his teeth when he talked. The smallest things are often the ones that bother us the most, and the sound of silence was a huge deal to Barry.

One cause of tinnitus is TDS. Other causes are exposure to loud noises, chronic ear infections, head injuries, and viral infections. These types of tinnitus generally don't improve with only testosterone replacement. However, about 40 percent of tinnitus cases improve with testosterone. These patients also have other symptoms of TDS, and their tinnitus starts after age fifty.

It's thought that testosterone increases the fluid in the inner ear that buffers the sound of our heartbeat. We know that aging and low testosterone can cause the inner-ear canals to dry out. Testosterone is the great lubricator, and it rehydrates the inner ear just like it does the synovial fluid in the joints. With this lubrication, the high-pitched whine of TDS-induced tinnitus stops!

❑ Anxiety and Depression

Anxiety and depression occur more frequently when men experience TDS. Testosterone is a natural mood elevator, and the lack of it causes depression in most men. But many men avoid dealing with their depression. They self-medicate with alcohol or get prescription drugs for their symptoms. But these remedies don't treat the *cause* of the problem. Replacing testosterone can reduce anxiety and depression levels in men without the need to self-medicate.

Bill, the CEO of a computer software company, came to see me because whenever he had to make a presentation to his board, or give speeches to the community, or film a commercial—all things he had done regularly and smoothly in the past—he suffered from disturbing surges of anxiety. He went to his physician and asked for medication to control his anxiety attacks. He hated the idea of taking these medicines, but he was desperate. The drugs made him sluggish and tired, and he knew he couldn't run his company like that. So he stopped taking them and continued to suffer. Each time he was just a bit nervous he began to perspire, his heart raced, and he couldn't control his anxiety.

Then he heard me speak on a local radio show about how the onset of anxiety attacks in men over forty is often due to testosterone loss. He immediately made an appointment to see me without even discussing it with his wife, which is not uncommon for men.

When Bill met with me, he said that he hoped his symptoms had a physical root and weren't a sign of weakness or a defect of character. His identity was very closely tied to his masculinity, determination, and strength of will power. We found he had, indeed, lost free T, which had caused surges of the pituitary hormones LH and FSH, giving him anxiety attacks.

Bill decided to try testosterone pellets. Within four months, he no longer had anxiety attacks and his depression had lifted. In addition, his sense of sexuality and his sexual performance were better than they'd been in years. Like most men, he was reluctant to admit that this miracle was the result of testosterone pellets alone. But he was impressed that he was saving more than the cost of his other doctor visits and the other medicines he'd been taking, and he had none of the side effects he'd had with antidepressants and antianxiety drugs.

In most cases, mood disorders can't be attributed solely to hormonal deficiency. When anxiety and depression appear after age forty in men, low T is usually one of the causes; however, there are other mood problems that are unrelated to low-T. Bipolar disorder, long-term depression, and generalized anxiety disorder are usually present long before age forty.

Conditions that existed before testosterone levels fell won't improve by taking testosterone. Patients who have been on antidepressants or antipsychotics should stay on them when they start testosterone until their prescribing physician determines they've improved enough to decrease their dose or be weaned off the medication. This doesn't always happen for men with long-term mood illnesses.

There is, however, a characteristic type of anxiety that men experience when their testosterone drops. Surges in their LH and FSH result in anxiety attacks that they've never experienced before. This is how the pituitary reacts to low levels of testosterone.

Most male patients describe their anxiety in the same way. Their attacks last a few minutes; they come in surges and are worse at night, when they drink alcohol, and when they are under stress—the same conditions that cause hot flashes in women. When their testosterone pellets produce an adequate, normal, young, and healthy free T blood level, these symptoms stop right away. It's the same physiologic response to low estrogen in women, but men experience low free T in a different way. The LH and FSH surges in men don't cause hot flashes; they cause anxiety attacks.

Depression is a bit different. Depression increases as men age due to the loss of testosterone, which decreases endorphins, serotonin levels, and the other neurotransmitters such as dopamine that provide us with a good mood.

Unfortunately, most men are placed on antidepressants or antianxiety agents for these symptoms when what they really need is to have their testosterone replaced. These medications may superficially help the emotional symptoms, but they don't generally bring these men back to normal. Plus, the side effects of these drugs cause loss of libido and ED. It's the wrong solution to the problem. The right solution solves the *cause* of the problem, not just the *symptoms* of the problem.

Sean, a forty-five-year-old man, and his wife came to see me. It was his wife's idea. She said that over the past four years, Sean had become a "lump" at home. He used to go out after work to play ball with the kids or work in the yard. On Saturdays, he'd play tennis or golf with his buddies, but now he didn't do any of that.

Sean said nothing was wrong and he was just tired. He didn't want to have sex because he was "just tired." The kids didn't energize him the way they did before, but he felt sure that he'd get over it. His wife feared that his lack of mojo could cause him to lose his job.

Sean reported that work was going well, but that it took all his energy to get up and go to work every day. At his wife's urging, he'd gone to his doctor to ask for an antidepressant. He'd tried these antidepressants for three months but didn't feel they were helping. He noticed that since he'd begun taking them, he didn't want to have sex anymore at all! When he tried to perform to please his wife, it didn't work.

Sean didn't want to be depressed, nor did he want the label or the medicines or the side effects associated with antidepressants. He thought that if he could just rest for a while, things would get better. He wanted his wife and kids to be patient with him.

After the interview and his assessment, I showed Sean that both of his testosterone levels were low, and I encouraged him to try testosterone pellets. He was reluctant to have yet more medicine, so I suggested that he try a single treatment to see if it made a difference. If he didn't like it, there would be no lasting effect from having tried pellets. However, if he felt more energized, more sexual, more alert, and stronger, he might want to continue with the pellets.

Sean came to see me five months after his first pellet insertion, and he seemed somewhat better. His motivation and focus were still bad. He had been weaned off his antidepressants and now his sex life was great, but what was the answer to his remaining problems?

In my discussion with the couple, I learned that Sean had been treated for ADD as a child. As an adult, he'd quit taking the medicines and taught himself compensatory strategies to mitigate the concentration and focus problems that are signs of ADD. I encouraged him to revisit this decision after he'd been on testosterone replacement to determine if having the correct medicines for ADD, in addition to having his testosterone replaced, would bring him back to normal.

Because pellets create a passive on-demand reservoir in the body, Sean's history of noncompliance and resistance didn't recur. After he had a couple of pellet treatments, we discussed medication for his ADD. Sean listened to my recommendation, and he agreed to try an ADD medication.

Bingo! Treating his ADD plus taking T pellets was the answer, and Sean ultimately had a happy ending.

❑ **Man Boobs**

Have you ever watched the Senior Golf Tour and seen the players—all over age fifty—walk down the fairway with their man boobs bouncing up and down? You have to wonder how these great golfers let themselves get in such shape. They have money, they have fame, and they have marketing people buffing up their image all the time, but still they do nothing about this unsightly appearance.

If you think the reason these intelligent athletes don't use modern medicine to shrink their man boobs is because it's against the Senior PGA rules to use testosterone and Arimidex®, then you might be surprised. The Senior PGA doesn't test its players for drugs. Sadly, testosterone replacement is still considered a "dangerous drug" by the Drug Enforcement Administration, even though all humans produce it. The Senior PGA is probably the smartest sport association because it doesn't restrict the use of testosterone replacement for their aging professionals. And yet, their players apparently still consider testosterone replacement to be a crutch rather than the path to good health.

Getting man boobs is not a certain destiny for all men, but most men transform more and more of their testosterone into estrogen every year, with these results:

- Estrogen uses up more of the available testosterone and turns it into estrone and estradiol, which stimulate man boobs.

- Estrogen binds up the free testosterone, decreasing the active testosterone available for male sexuality.

The answer to man boobs is the drug Arimidex®, an aromatase inhibitor that blocks the conversion of testosterone into estrogen. For men over fifty who have low total T and low free T, replacement is necessary, and pellets are the most effective way to administer testosterone. And it's critical to achieve fat loss by any means possible. Together, these three steps make it possible to lose man boobs, as well as release more available free testosterone.

If you already have man boobs, then *do not use testosterone gel or patches*. Sixty percent to eighty percent of those forms of testosterone convert into estrogen as they pass through the skin.

However, if you already have man boobs, then *do not use testosterone gel or patches*. Sixty percent to eighty percent of those forms of testosterone convert into estrogen as they pass through the skin.

If you make plenty of total testosterone, then weight loss and Arimidex® (anastrozole) may be all you need to lose your man boobs. *Never consent to surgery until you have used these methods first!*

❏ Smaller Genitals

Men who are well-endowed, or are normally endowed at any size, aren't happy when their genitals get smaller as they age. Their genitals not only shrink at rest, but without testosterone, blood flow is not as it once was in their youth. Therefore, even when erect, a man's penis doesn't grow to its previous size. And even worse for a man, after a while, if testosterone is insufficient, the penis and testes shrink permanently. They won't return to their previous size without testosterone replacement.

This aging type of shrinkage isn't like the "Seinfeld shrinkage" that George experienced when he went swimming in cold water. It's a semipermanent smaller size of the penis and the testicles—while at rest and when stimulated. The drugs Viagra® and Cialis® can increase the penis size by increasing vascular dilation, which fills the penis with blood, but it doesn't last. Without testosterone, youthful size of the male penis can't be replicated.

Testosterone stimulates penis growth while at rest and when "at attention," and it brings most men of any age back to their younger, healthy size—like when they were in their thirties. A new partner may not see any difference in you, because men are naturally individual in their nonaroused as well as aroused sizes; however, a partner who's been with you for a long time will certainly notice. Whether it bothers them or not is also individual.

Even without long-term partners, men are always "out there" in bathrooms, locker rooms, and other settings in which they compare themselves to other men. There's nothing in a woman's experience that can compare to this, but I have an idea of how important penis size is to men. They tell me frequently about being disappointed with their diminished anatomy.

There seems to be some confusion about what happens to a man's genitals when he takes testosterone. I'm often asked by my patients if their penis, "dick," "Johnson," or whatever you want to call it will shrink if they take testosterone. Of course, the answer is no. The male member is usually brought back to pre-TDS size within a few months of replacing testosterone. Hearing this is always reassuring to my patients.

The next thing I tell men prior to their T replacement is that when a man takes testosterone, just like when he ages, his testicles will shrink. When your testes stop making their own T, they begin to shrink. This is a natural outcome. When we replace

T with pellets, it shuts down the T production from the testes. After T replacement, you don't need your testes to produce T because with the pellets, you get the benefits you once got from your testes.

This is OK for some men but unacceptable to others. As for how women feel about shrinking testes, my personal survey found that the size of the scrotum isn't a concern for women one way or another.

For men who are worried about a shrinking scrotum, I offer a twice-weekly, self-administered injection of HCG to keep the testes stimulated and normal-sized. If this makes a man feel normal and desirable, then he should get that treatment along with his testosterone pellet replacement. I believe what's good for one sex is good for the other, and hundreds of thousands of women have had breast implants for similar reasons!

❏ Feeling Old and Near the End of Life

When you don't feel well and are depressed, exhausted, and unmotivated, your quality of life is diminished. Days drag by and the end of life seems near. As we age, we sometimes think back to those things that we'll never see again: the graduation of a child or grandchild, the last ten springs or summers ... you know what I mean. All of a sudden, life has an end point and you're racing toward it.

It's not just that a man *is* getting older, it's that he *feels* old. Feeling old is a symptom of low testosterone. The aching, the wrinkles, and all the symptoms we've talked about make a man feel really old and helpless—and there's nothing worse for a man than feeling helpless!

There are two treatments for feeling old and displaying all the signs of aging: first, take testosterone and, second, find a purpose. When we feel good, we have many options that we couldn't even consider before, and many men start the second chapter of their life with a new job, an invention, or a new partner. In the twenty-first century, we will probably live for eighty to ninety-five years, which means there are thirty to forty-five years left to live after the average onset of TDS. With testosterone, this third of life has many possibilities to explore.

❑ More Body Hair but Less Head Hair

Many men over age fifty complain to me about how hairy they've gotten. They have hair where they never had it before: upper arms, back, chest, ears, and nose. And while the hair on their bodies has grown, the hair on their head has thinned. I reassure them that replacing their lost testosterone with pellets won't increase their body hair or receding hair line. In fact, in some men, body hair decreases.

As most men get older, they make more DHT (dihydrotestosterone) and *that* hormone causes both increased body hair and hair loss on the head. As you age, the balance between your T and DHT switches. When T is high, you can grow a rich, thick head of hair. As you switch to more DHT and less T, the hair production on your head is impacted as a result of increased DHT. As we regulate this balance between T and DHT using pellet treatment, we can help stabilize the amount of hair on your head.

One way to decrease head hair loss is by using a drug called *finasteride* (sold under the brand names Propecia® and Proscar®), which decreases the conversion of testosterone to DHT. It doesn't work for all men, but I assure you that testosterone in pellet form makes the least DHT of all T replacements.

Even if men come to us after five years has passed since their hair loss became obvious, most can stop the loss with pellet testosterone. Finasteride helps many of them reduce DHT, which helps manage their body hair and slows the hair loss on their head, too.

There is, however, a negative side effect of taking finasteride. For many men, finasteride decreases DHT to such a low level that they don't feel the positive benefits of testosterone. It's a balancing act, and you need the right doctor to help you balance the scales.

❑ New Migraine Headaches

Vascular swelling in the brain causes headaches, nausea, pain on one side of the head, sensitivity to light, and sometimes vomiting—and it's often incapacitating. It's not unheard of for men to experience migraine headaches, but when their testosterone levels drop below optimal levels, they experience them more often. Men are at risk for this type of migraine—the hormonal migraine—in midlife and thereafter.

Testosterone plays a role in neurologic stability by modulating neurotransmitters and brain hormones. If there's an imbalance that triggers a migraine, testosterone will balance it so the migraine doesn't occur. Testosterone is also important in vascular stability Remember, it treats inflammation. The presence of testosterone prevents the swelling of intracranial veins that increase pressure in the brain and cause the incapacitating symptoms of migraine headaches.

To determine if you have hormonal migraine headaches, check the boxes below that match your experience.

<u>Signs of Hormonal Migraines:</u>

❑ Abrupt onset of one-sided head pain

❑ Sensitivity to light

❑ Seeing bright spots (aura) before the pain starts

❑ Onset after the age of fifty

❑ Nausea with the headache

❑ Does not begin in your forehead and neck

❑ Is stimulated by stress

If you have three or more of the above symptoms, then you may have a vascular migraine that can be treated with testosterone pellets. But first, a headache workup must be done to make sure that you aren't having symptoms from more severe medical diagnoses like a stroke, blood clot, or brain tumor. Your neurologist or your primary care physician should do a complete physical exam that includes measuring your blood pressure and pulse, an EKG, an MRI of your brain and/or an EEG, and a carotid Doppler ultrasound so he or she can rule out dangerous medical conditions.

Next, rule out other types of headaches. The other headaches that can be confused with migraines include.

Other Types of Headaches:
- Allergy headaches
- Sinus headaches
- High blood pressure headaches
- Muscle-spasm tension headaches
- TMJ headache—temporo-mandibular headache from gritting your teeth
- Tooth pain

The above types of headaches can't be treated with testosterone. Allergy headaches can be diagnosed by tracking your history of headaches to see if they occur each year at the same time of year when certain plants are producing pollen. If you'd like a medical diagnosis of your allergies, you can do a battery of allergy tests. If allergies are the problem, then treating them with allergy medicine or allergy shots should be tried. Testosterone is *not* the treatment for these headaches.

Sinus headaches are easy to diagnose: if you tap your cheeks and/or forehead and it hurts, it's not a migraine, it's a sinus headache. You should see your primary care physician or an ENT doctor to treat your infected or clogged sinuses.

Diagnosing high blood pressure headaches requires taking your blood pressure every time you have a headache. If your blood pressure is low or normal, your blood pressure isn't the source of your pain. If it's high—above 150/90—you'll need to be evaluated to determine if your blood pressure elevation is really the cause or effect of your pain. Sometimes this pain causes an increase in blood pressure; and other times high blood pressure can cause headaches. Testosterone is not the answer.

Muscle-spasm headaches are always on both sides of the head, and they start in your neck, shoulders, and forehead. They are not unilateral (on one side of the head). They should be treated with massage, heat, and muscle relaxants. Testosterone is not the answer.

You need to see a dentist for both TMJ and tooth pain. TMJ is the unconscious gritting of your teeth during sleep and stress, and tooth pain can be caused by infection or an abscess. Both can cause a severe headache and need specialized treatment from your dentist.

Migraines that are initiated by low testosterone levels get worse as time goes by, and they immediately disappear when testosterone levels return to normal. This symptom of low T shouldn't be ignored. It could be something worse, and ruling out other causes of headache could save your life. You don't want to just assume that your migraines are due to low T; it could be something life-threatening.

❏ Thinning Skin

Men's testosterone levels are many times higher than women's during the first half of their lives. Male testosterone levels cause their skin to be more elastic, thicker, and more taut than women's—until they start losing testosterone as they age.

As men's free testosterone level drops, their skin becomes less elastic, thinner, and sags in places it never sagged before (upper arms, jowls, and thighs). In some men over age seventy, the skin becomes paper thin.

If testosterone creams or gels are applied, these symptoms of aging are not altered. Testosterone pellet replacement is key to recovering normal skin thickness and oil production, which keeps skin taught and hydrated. Great skin requires a young, healthy male level of testosterone; a diet rich in protein and omega 3 and omega 6 fatty acids; and good twice-daily face cleansing.

❑ Frequent Urination / Enlarged Prostate

"I can't believe I'm telling you this," Sam, a fifty-five-year-old, well-dressed patient said to me at his first consultation in my office. "My worst symptom of low T is that I spend my day locating bathrooms so I can pee, and then I can go only a little bit. When I think I'm done, I zip up, and I go a little more and leave a stain on my trousers. I can't live like this!

"My urologist says my prostate is enlarged, and he acts like this is normal. I'm in my fifties! Whenever I bring it up, he changes the subject to avoid this issue. This is a real problem! I'm a salesman and I run around in my car all the time; so I can't always find a bathroom when I need it. My urologist hasn't done anything for me. What do you *have in your bag of tricks?"*

As men age, they often complain of frequent urination—a problem that begins to control their lives. Sam's condition was worse than most, but many men find they can't drive as far as they used to without stopping for a restroom break. Or they don't get much sleep because they have to get up multiple times per night to urinate. Others can't hold it when they need to go and have trouble with leakage and dribbling. Luckily, testosterone treatment plus some medication can treat these symptoms.

These symptoms are caused by the growth of the prostate gland. Three factors change in men that stimulate the growth of the prostate: lower free T levels; elevation of the T by-product, DHT; and increase in estrone. One or all three of these changes can increase the size of the prostate gland and result in the symptoms that Sam experienced.

There are medicines that men can take to relieve these symptoms. Others help slow prostate enlargement and reduce the negative impact on men. These meds include Flomax®—whose generic equivalent is tamsulosin—which enhances the starting and stopping of urine flow and decreases dribbling; finasteride—also called Proscar® and Propecia®—which decreases the level of DHT and helps shrink the prostate (fertile women are not supposed to touch this, so be careful how you store and take it); and dutasteride, which works like finasteride to shrink the prostate by decreasing the DHT levels.

There are side effects to these drugs. Finasteride and dutasteride cause a reduction in the volume of ejaculate. This reduction does not impact your ability to enjoy an orgasm, but you or your partner may notice this change and be concerned about it. It doesn't result in any dangerous problems. A fourth drug, Arimidex®, can be used to decrease estrone and, therefore, the size of the prostate.

These medicines are all effective for the specific symptoms that accompany prostate enlargement, and some may be necessary—even if testosterone pellets are used—to actually treat the problem. It depends on how long a man has had symptoms of prostate enlargement.

In some cases, a very large prostate will require surgery performed by a urologist. Many men call the procedure "roto-rooter surgery," but officially it's called a TURP (transurethral resection of the prostate). This procedure effectively reduces the frequency of urination, incontinence, and difficulty starting and stopping a stream of urine. But one risk is incontinence and/or trouble ending the flow of urine. You should follow your urologist's advice if this procedure is recommended for you. You can still replace your testosterone with pellets after the procedure is completed.

Quiz: How Many Symptoms Do You Have?

Return to the first page of this chapter and check each symptom that you have. If you have three or more symptoms, the next step is to have your blood drawn and evaluated by an expert. In the next chapter, you'll learn about the blood tests that diagnose TDS and what is needed to make a diagnosis.

Remember, every man is an individual, and the amount of testosterone that he needs is unique to him. Blood levels tell only one side of the story. Your symptoms, your lab results, and your physical signs together determine whether you will benefit from treatment.

The checklist is meant primarily for men to use as a guideline and then see their doctor to evaluate if their symptoms are due to a loss of testosterone. My experience is that replacing testosterone is often the most critical and least-expensive intervention to bring you back to good health and help you avoid many of the common illnesses and conditions of aging. My goal is for you to have a long and healthy life with total independence and functionality.

CHAPTER 3

Do You Have Any of the Diseases or Conditions of Aging? Testosterone Can Help!

- ❏ Insulin Resistance
- ❏ Adult-Onset Diabetes
- ❏ Obesity
- ❏ High Cholesterol, Triglycerides, or Inflammation
- ❏ Parkinson's Disease
- ❏ Osteoporosis
- ❏ Autoimmune Diseases
- ❏ Dementia and Alzheimer's Disease
- ❏ Male Breast Cancer
- ❏ Cancer
- ❏ Sarcopenia
- ❏ Risk of Early Mortality

One of the most important actions we can take to prevent future diseases in men is to replace their testosterone when it becomes deficient. Hundreds of studies show that low T levels increase the risk of getting one of the following diseases: Alzheimer's disease, Parkinson's disease, heart disease, stroke, adult-onset diabetes, autoimmune diseases, male breast cancer, and cancer of all other kinds. Almost as many studies prove that replacing testosterone can *delay* or *prevent* those same diseases in men as they age, but most men at the age of onset of testosterone deficiency symptoms haven't heard this news.

I don't understand why all doctors don't recommend that men choose testosterone replacement when the evidence is so compelling that testosterone helps avoid disease. It seems that keeping men healthy as they age isn't a priority in our medical community, but I'm determined to make it *your* personal priority. I wrote this book to save men from the diseases of aging, so they can live full, vibrant, and virile lives.

> **If you don't yet have the disease yourself but have a family history of one of these diseases—or if you have a precondition leading to one of these diseases—then you can possibly delay or prevent the disease with testosterone pellets.**

If you already have one of these diseases, receiving testosterone pellets can help treat or reverse that disease. If you don't yet have the disease but have a family history of one of these diseases—or if you have a precondition leading to one of these diseases—then you can possibly delay or prevent the disease with testosterone pellets.

What Does High Risk Mean?

There's a big difference between having a high risk of developing a disease and actually getting that disease. We can't change risk factors that are inherited from our parents, and there's little we can do about the environmental risks from chemicals that seep into our water and food supply that change our genetics and make us sick. An individual can't change these by himself; only society can. But you *can* alter the risk factors that have to do with lifestyle, such as smoking, excessive drinking, and overeating. And by replacing testosterone during the first ten years after TDS begins, you can avoid or mitigate many of the diseases listed on page 63.

Genetic Risk Assessment

Thanks to affordable genetic testing, genetic risks have become more and more identifiable. We can learn of our genetic weaknesses and risk factors, and stop worrying about diseases that we have no risk for. Remember, having a gene for a disease doesn't mean you will get that disease. It means that you're more likely to get it than someone who doesn't have that gene. Knowledge of your genetics allows you to take the necessary steps to avoid getting diseases that run in your family.

I always ask my patients about their family history and the countries of origin of their ancestors. This information helps me appreciate the inborn risks of each individual patient. It helps my diagnosis if they have done a cheek swab with 23 and Me, National Geo, or Ancestry.com to find the countries from which they inherit their genes, as well as telling me which diseases run in their families. I also ask what diseases they have had in the past or currently, which often will change my medical management of that individual.

Not all diseases are more common as men age. People of any age are susceptible to communicable diseases like viruses and some cancers, especially blood cancers and sarcoma. The diseases of aging are just that—diseases that are rarely experienced by people under age fifty.

We used to see that men began to lose their T after age fifty. Now we're seeing more and more men who are experiencing this loss in their forties. We don't know why, but even while we look for that answer, we still recognize that the best intervention is the replacement of the lost T.

Our modern environment and lifestyle have lowered the age at which men experience symptoms and diseases of low testosterone (diseases of aging). Now men are dealing with these diseases almost a decade earlier than men did a generation ago.

What specific factors of modern life cause early TDS and the diseases of aging? Here are some factors that have caused men to lose the ability to make adequate testoserone at an earlier age than in the past.

<u>Causes of Early Testosterone Loss:</u>

- Less exercise in daily routine
- More constant psychological stress
- More simple sugars in our diet
- Less nutrition in our food
- Drastic increase in endocrine-disrupting chemicals in the last twenty years (such as in plastics)
- Higher average weight for the male population
- Heavy alcohol intake

Most of these lifestyle changes have been creeping up on us over the last thirty to forty years, and our government hasn't helped prevent them as it should. In fact, government at all levels has been part of our problem. Public education has changed to cut out physical activity. We've deleted gym and recess from many public schools. The government told mothers how to feed their children using the Food Pyramid, based on cereals and sugar, so we fed our children more and more carbohydrates, which triggered an epidemic of adult-onset diabetes and obesity. We're now programmed to crave carbs, and now we have a national health crisis based on the fact that almost half of Americans are obese and have adult-onset diabetes.

However, it's not all about the government. Our fresh food has lost much of its nutritious value due to overfarming the land without replacing the minerals and nutrients we need for our food to be healthy. Eating fresh food is always better than eating processed food, but an apple today doesn't contain the same nutrition as an apple did in 1959.

Last but not least, industrialization and consumerism have caused pervasive pollution by chemicals called environmental disrupting chemicals (EDCs), which affect human and animal hormones. EDCs are those chemicals in plastics and pesticides that act as antihormones—or estrogens—in the human body. They are all man-made. The use of plastics has made our lives more convenient, but at what cost? The by-products of plastic production are invisible but are now firmly embedded in our food sources, air, and water, causing obesity and illness.

EDCs are hard to track until they accumulate in the human body. In the male body, they act as estrogens and cause development of belly fat and man boobs, which decreases circulating testosterone. The decline of testosterone levels in the American male will eventually affect fertility and the ability to procreate. This is a real threat and one from which we have no known protection.

My treatment plan is to replace and supplement testosterone in men as soon as their testosterone levels become deficient as a method of counteracting the forces of EDCs in our environment. It's not a cure, but it will undo some of the damage that EDCs do.

Due to modern life, men fall below the critical healthy level of testosterone in their late thirties and early forties, rather than their fifties. In fact, the total and free testosterone levels of most men under fifty have dropped to an unhealthy level. In turn, the diseases of aging occur at an earlier and earlier age. Every year it gets worse, and younger men experience symptoms of TDS. Changes in lifestyle and testosterone replacement are the only tools we currently have to combat this increasing problem.

The total and free testosterone levels of most men under fifty have dropped to an unhealthy level. In turn, the diseases of aging occur at an earlier and earlier age.

❏ Insulin Resistance

Insulin resistance (IR) is a precursor to adult-onset diabetes mellitus and is often called *hypoglycemia*. It's a genetic- and hormone-regulated imbalance characterized by the inefficient use of blood sugar for energy. IR makes it impossible to use the food we eat to make enough energy for us to live. Rather than create energy, we make fat and put stress on our pancreas at the same time. When we eat carbohydrates, our insulin production overreacts, and we get low blood sugar (hypoglycemia) a few hours later. The emergence of this condition depends on an individual's genetic risk for Adult-Onset Diabetes and his history of eating a high-carbohydrate diet without adequate exercise.

The symptoms of IR include persistent weight gain that is unresponsive to decreasing calories eaten, an increase in abdominal fat, and fatigue a few hours after eating simple carbs or high-volume, carbohydrate-dominant meals. The more processed sugar and carbohydrates a man takes in on a regular basis, the worse his IR becomes.

Here's what happens when you have IR. When you eat a carbohydrate-rich meal, you stimulate the pancreas to overproduce insulin. Insulin is meant to piggyback blood sugar into the cells, where sugar is turned into energy and heat. If you make too much insulin every time you eat, your insulin surges and the cells at the end of the line become resistant and won't allow the insulin plus blood sugar "package" in. This causes the blood sugar to "bounce off" the cells and deposit it as fat. The blood sugar level in your blood dramatically drops because no energy is being created, and you become fatigued, tired, and sleepy. This is hypoglycemia. When you eat something "carby" again, the cycle recurs.

Over time, you build up so much fat that the insulin you produce can't service all the body's needs, and your blood sugar begins to rise and remains high. That is *adult-onset diabetes*.

Low T levels result in more severe hypoglycemia and greater insulin resistance. If you replace testosterone to young, healthy levels, you can reverse IR and lose weight if you follow a low-carb diet and exercise. If you don't, it's a never-ending cycle of weight gain and fatigue, ending in diabetes.

❏ **Adult-Onset Diabetes**

If you replace testosterone to young, healthy levels, you can reverse IR and lose weight if you follow a low-carb diet and exercise.

Diabetes that occurs later in life and is associated with obesity is called Adult-Onset Diabetes Mellitus (AODM), or type 2 diabetes. It's become *the* epidemic of the twenty-first century. Over half of the men whose bloodwork I've reviewed have undiagnosed AODM or prediabetes with elevated triglycerides and elevated glucose. But they aren't yet at the level of outright AODM. All these men have low free testosterone, elevated estrone (>30) and/or estradiol levels (>40), and most have low DHT (dihydrotestosterone). The associated symptoms of men with low T and AODM include fatigue, belly fat gain, weight gain, loss of muscle, hunger, and addiction to alcohol or sugar.

If AODM is not treated with testosterone and an insulin sensitizer such as metformin, it almost invariably leads to erectile dysfunction, heart disease, stroke, and eventually death. Diabetes tortures you and then kills you.

In my first conversation with a new patient, I always review his lifestyle—exercise, diet, alcohol, drug use, and family history. Most men who have both low T and AODM or prediabetes want to know why they have this combined problem. The answer is surprisingly straightforward. Over time, as T decreases with age, men become insulin-resistant, which causes fatigue and hypoglycemia. Hypoglycemia leads to craving carbs to feel better, which increases weight gain and belly fat and makes the problem worse. In addition, more belly fat makes estrogens—estrone and estradiol—which bind testosterone up, inactivating it and decreasing its production, which in turn further reduces testosterone levels and causes a man to gain weight and make more estrogen.

Both IR and low T must be addressed for a man to break free from this cycle. Testosterone must be replaced in a non-oral, nontransdermal way, either by intramuscular shots of depo-testosterone or subcutaneous pellets. Insulin resistance must be treated with a drug called metformin (an insulin sensitizer), a low-carb diet, and daily aerobic exercise. Patient compliance is vital to success. Ideally, when a man reaches a youthful muscle mass and weight for his height, the testosterone supplementation will continue, but metformin and other medications for diabetes can be stopped.

Barry is a forty-two-year-old heating and cooling business owner who has gained sixty pounds since he was thirty-six. He complains that no matter what he does, he can't lose weight. He continues to gain belly fat. Not only has this made him miserable, but he's so tired after he eats that he has to take a nap in his office at work. Because of his low testosterone and weight gain, his knees are killing him, so he doesn't walk or work out anymore. He might have to have knee replacements. Most upsetting to him is that he has ED that is not completely resolved by taking Viagra®. He said he was a "once-a-day man" when it came to sex, and now he is barely having sex once a week. His wife of twenty years thinks he's having an affair because he doesn't desire her anymore. Barry was desperate to get better. I'd be remiss if I didn't mention here that while ED can be caused by low testosterone, ED is also recognized as an early warning sign for heart attack and stroke. I reminded Barry if he failed at this treatment, he'd be at risk for AODM, heart disease, and knee replacements in the near future. His father had the same issues, and he remembered how his dad had become so frustrated and angry that he withdrew from the world because of his pain and obesity.

I put Barry on Dr. Maupin's Low-Carb Diet and banned him from sugared soda, juices, and all baked goods. He had type O blood, so I told him to eat red meat and all the fruit and vegetables he wanted. He had to cut out beer, but when he got to his ideal weight, he could slowly add back moderate drinking—no more than two beers per day. This was his forever eating plan; it was not a diet.

We inserted testosterone pellets with Arimidex® to replace his low T. The Arimidex® would decrease estrogen conversion from testosterone. I also told him to exercise daily using a recumbent bike, so he wouldn't further damage his knees. Because he was to bike forty-five minutes a day, he put his bike in his office. He also took several supplements daily, including DIM to decrease belly fat, berberine to stabilize blood sugars, and arginine and ornithine to increase muscle mass. He promised to follow the plan and return in four months.

At his follow-up visit, Barry was a changed man! He looked more like his chronological age and had lost the swollen look he had before. He said it was easy to eat right after he talked to his wife about what was going on. She got on board with the program right away and made sure that he ate properly. She also cleared the pantry of sugary, processed junk food.

Barry is on his way and, by the way, he is again a "once-a-day man!" He now knows what life could be like if he stops leading a healthy life. I believe that he'll continue to work toward optimum health now that he knows the cause of his problems and how to fix them.

❑ Obesity

Obesity has reached epidemic proportions in the US. It's caused by some of the same factors that cause AODM, and often ends in the development of diabetes—sometimes insulin-dependent diabetes. However, there are some risk factors for obesity that are *different* from the causes of diabetes.

<u>Risk Factors That Lead to Obesity, Other Than Diabetes:</u>

- Genetic predispositions that prevent you from feeling full
- Genetic mutations that make you hungry all the time
- Genetic predispositions for obesity
- Genetic code for insulin resistance
- Childhood conditioning to use food to feel good
- Poor eating habits taught from childhood

- Lack of exercise
- Low growth hormone and testosterone since puberty

How does low T change the body mechanisms that result in obesity? Like falling dominos, one hormone deficit results in weight gain, which stimulates insulin, which stimulates more weight gain. It's a cycle that continues until death, ever increasing fat production over time.

It's not just the accumulation of fat in the testosterone-deprived body that causes a man to become obese. Without testosterone, a man loses muscle every day. The muscle is replaced by fat, and because of that, he doesn't burn as many calories. Day after day, his fat increases and the largest calorie-burning system in the human body—his musculature—shrinks, which causes his metabolism to further decrease.

This is why weight lifting is a good first step to increase your metabolism, even in the face of low T. After testosterone replacement, weight-bearing exercise is the best boost for regaining a faster metabolism.

There's another problem with fat in the abdomen, which is generally where men carry it. Fat that's centered in the abdomen increases both estrogens *and* insulin. Estrogens, such as estradiol and estrone, decrease the amount of free T, which shrinks muscles and steals energy while increasing arterial plaque production. Insulin increases when weight is gained, so every year you gain five to ten pounds, you increase your risk of diabetes and heart disease.

You can stop the perpetual obesity cycle by combining four things: testosterone pellets, metformin, weight lifting, and a low-carb diet.

You can stop the perpetual obesity cycle by combining four things: testosterone pellets, metformin, weight lifting, and a low-carb diet. Try it. You'll look and feel younger, while saving yourself from heart attack, diabetes, and all the misery these diseases create.

❏ High Cholesterol, Triglycerides, and Inflammation

When I woke up from my hypoxic event after my hysterectomy in 2002, I was in the ICU on a respirator. I had no idea what had happened. All I could think was that I'd had a heart attack or stroke. Because I could think, I figured it was probably a heart attack and that my life as I knew it would be over! I'd never run, ski, ride a bike, or hike up mountains on vacation. I thought about my teenage daughter and the fact that I might not be able to work! It's true that your life flies in front of you as you're on the verge of death. I know what a heart attack and heart failure can do. I've seen it.

I didn't want to suffer that, and I asked God to take me home. It happened in a flash, and I was almost there, prostrate at the feet of Christ and unbelievably healthy and happy. I really wanted to stay, but I was told to come back to my earthly family, and BAM! I was back. However, God did answer my prayers. I had not had a heart attack, but an anesthetic complication that caused the doctors to fear that I'd have severe brain damage. My Lithuanian mother and Italian father always told me I was a "tough cookie," and they were right; I was created of true, strong peasant stock. I recovered and followed God's direction to use testosterone pellet therapy to save other people's lives!

Dr. Kathy Maupin

I tell you that story because I want you to know how afraid I was of having a heart attack. I knew that after one, my life would never be the same, and I'd face a long period of physical recuperation. Instead, the biggest factor in my treatment and recovery has been taking testosterone and estradiol pellets. My heart does have an arrhythmia, but nothing else is wrong. There was *no damage* to my heart muscle, which is highly unusual. I have my full life back. I eat right, exercise, am at my ideal weight, and will never risk having a heart attack if I can help it.

They say that high cholesterol is the primary culprit in heart disease and atherosclerosis, but I'll tell you a secret: the newest finding—that will become standard in the next five years—is that it's not cholesterol or high-cholesterol foods, but *inflammation* plus *carbohydrates* that leads to heart attacks!

❏ Parkinson's Disease

Parkinson's disease is a progressive neurological disorder of the part of the brain that produces dopamine, a neurotransmitter that allows us to experience joy, make facial expressions, have quickness of movement, and enjoy restful sleep. Parkinson's disease usually begins after the age of sixty and is more common in men than women. It starts with an onset of tremors of the hands and face, then progresses to include poor balance, lack of facial movements, fatigue, depression, a slow gait, insomnia, and, finally, the inability to think.

We know how the disease progresses and what it looks like, but we don't know what triggers it or turns it on. As with many other degenerative diseases of old age, the trigger may be low free testosterone levels.

When Parkinson's occurs in men who are genetically at risk, the downward cycle begins and the symptoms can vary in acceleration. Parkinson's disease generally ends in death after an unrelenting progression of worsening symptoms.

Testosterone is the hormone of regeneration, and that includes regenerating the cells of the brain, as well as bones, skin, blood vessels, and muscle mass.

Testosterone is the hormone of regeneration, and that includes regenerating the cells of the brain, as well as bones, skin, blood vessels, and muscle mass. When we age without testosterone, we're generally in a catabolic state: more cells die than are replaced with new cells, which explains loss of bone and muscle mass, brain shrinkage, skin that hangs off the limbs and face, diminished height, and loss of intellectual capacity.

In the case of Parkinson's, the brain cells in the area of the *substantia nigra* that produce dopamine begin to die and aren't replaced. This cell death results in fewer brain cells to make dopamine and, therefore, lower levels of the neurotransmitter that does so much for us. Testosterone supplementation is the first treatment for Parkinson's that may actually stop its progression and even remedy many of the accompanying changes. It's gratifying to follow my patients with Parkinson's who receive testosterone and witness their improvements.

> **Testosterone supplementation is the first treatment for Parkinson's that may actually stop its progression and even remedy many of the accompanying changes.**

Dan, my sixty-two-year-old patient, and his wife had travelled from another country to see me after none of the medications he was taking for Parkinson's had helped him. He was wasting away in body and soul, and it seemed as if a runaway train had taken over his health and his life!

His lovely wife had brought him to me, and at first sight, I thought I'd misunderstood his age. But I confirmed that he was, in fact, the same age as me, although he looked eighty-five, not sixty-two. He had lost most of his muscle mass and strength, and he could barely shuffle to walk into my office.

Dan's wife faithfully cared for him, and her pained face showed the wear and tear of caring for the love of her life who was disappearing before her eyes. She told me that Dan had been a lovely, handsome, driven man who'd managed a series of businesses in multiple countries for thirty years. He'd enjoyed a charmed life of golf and tennis, and he'd been a college football player. She said his progression from his diagnosis of Parkinson's to this point had been rapid, and she was trying everything she could to get him back to his former self.

I told them that he had very low total T and free T levels, and that testosterone therapy would not replace the drugs he was currently taking, so they shouldn't change any of his other medication at this time. I asked to see him again in five months after his first T pellet insertion.

Dan could only nod his head and speak a few words, but he was eager to start treatment. The only problem was figuring out how to insert the pellets in his emaciated body. He had lost all his fat and most of his muscle, and since T pellets can dissolve only in fat, we decided on a combined program of shots and pellets.

We began with Depo®-Testosterone (testosterone cypionate) shots every four weeks; because his wife was a nurse, she was able to administer them. We also placed pure testosterone pellets in the only pad of fat available on his body. I prayed that he would respond.

Six weeks later, I received an email from his wife. It was bittersweet because Dan was doing extremely well. But he'd developed a new problem; according to his wife, he was acting "schizophrenic"! He'd responded to the testosterone quickly and could now walk well, was more awake, and could think and interact easily with his wife and kids. He was so much better, but he'd become paranoid and was seeing things that weren't there.

When confronted with a confusing picture, I always go back to physiology. Here's what I knew: Dan was better, so he now had more dopamine than his Parkinson's drugs had been delivering when he was in my office. His muscles and peripheral nerves were improving, because he was walking better and faster than before. His sleep had improved, and his mind was sharp again. All this told me that the testosterone was working in the way it should. The "schizophrenia-like" problem was the glitch. A serious glitch.

Then I remembered that the neurotransmitter dopamine is typically very low in Parkinson's patients but very high in those with schizophrenia! Eureka! He was still taking his Parkinson's medications, which added dopamine to his system. This, coupled with the dopamine added by the increase in testosterone (one of the effects of the replacement of testosterone), had resulted in too much dopamine in Dan's system, which had led to his symptoms of schizophrenia. I asked his wife to call his prescribing doctor to get guidance on how to wean his medications down to the point where his schizophrenic-like symptoms disappeared but his Parkinson's was still treated.

My request to discuss his Parkinson's medication with his neurologist caused some difficulty. The doctor was unwilling to speak to me because, in all his years of treating Parkinson's, none of his patients had gotten better! He had never discussed the dosage of Parkinson's medicine he gave a patient with anyone before. Instead of asking what this miracle was, he was angry and would not engage. So Dan's wife weaned his meds down herself (she's a registered nurse), and he got so much better! While the situation was suboptimal, titrating down Dan's meds worked.

And the testosterone had worked. Dan is a changed man. He is gaining weight and strength daily, and he's acting more like himself.

I see changes like Dan experienced every day from administering a hormone replacement therapy that modern medicine has ignored. Perhaps this solution is being ignored by the broad medical community because there are glitzy, expensive, and innovative drugs to prescribe; however, they are unreasonably expensive, they don't work as well as T pellets, and they definitely don't bring patients with Parkinson's back to health. Dan's doctor had never seen a Parkinson's patient get better!

❑ Osteoporosis

Osteoporosis is a progressive thinning of the cortical bone layer around the outside circumference of all the bones of a body. It leads to fractures, disability, kyphosis (bent stature), vertebral collapse, spinal stenosis, chronic pain, and the inability to walk or heal after fractures. Osteopenia (thin bones that are not compromised enough to fracture without severe trauma) comes first and eventually progresses to osteoporosis, which means that simply stepping off a curb can cause a fracture.

Both osteoporosis and osteopenia are diagnosed by undergoing a low-dose X-ray called a bone-density test of the lower back vertebrae and the hip bone. We compare those results to the average bone density of a twenty-nine-year-old of the same sex. Sound absurd? If we compared your bone density to people of your current sex and age, we'd find that you might be average for your *age*, even if your bones were thin, because bones thin in everyone who doesn't receive testosterone—or estrogen in women as they age. We want to understand your bone density compared to a twenty-nine-year-old man, which is called your T-score. This is the same way we measure your hormone levels: we compare them to the average twenty- to forty-year-old man!

There are ten million people in the US, with osteoporosis, two million of whom are men. Osteoporosis usually worsens with age and it runs in families. People from northern Europe who also have a family history of osteoporosis have the highest genetic risk.

Genetically, people from areas nearer the equator have thicker bones. We used to think that osteoporosis was due to a lack of vitamin D and vitamin K2, but we now know that testosterone receptors are more sensitive in people from the lower latitudes; so similar blood free T levels provide thicker bones for people from countries near the equator.

Let's compare two people of the same sex, one from Sweden and another from Sicily. The Sicilian will have thicker bones than the Swede, even if their testosterone levels are the same. Those men and women from lower latitudes are much more sensitive to testosterone and do more with what they have.

Inherited, enviromental, and lifestyle factors decrease bone density.

Risk Factors for Osteoporosis:

- Old age
- Northern European heritage
- Intolerance to cow's milk
- Lack of exposure to sunlight
- Very thin body type and/or short stature
- Smoking
- Alcoholism
- Early testosterone deficiency and a lifelong low level of testosterone
- Brain damage to the pituitary or surgery that damages this gland
- Vitamin D and calcium deficiency
- Lack of weight-bearing exercise

- Use of corticosteroids
- Hyperthyroidism (overactive thyroid)
- Low growth hormone
- Elevated cortisol, adrenal hyperactivity, and stress
- Testosterone-blocking drugs, like treatment for prostate cancer (estrogen and finasteride)
- Removal of both testes because of cancer
- Drugs such as Propecia®, Lupron, amphetamines, cocaine, stimulants, drugs for autoimmune disease, and diuretics (not spironolactone)
- Damage to the testes from surgery, radiation, chemotherapy, or trauma to the scrotum

If you have three or more of these risk factors, please ask your primary care physician to order a bone-density test. This may prompt you to increase your testosterone blood level.

Osteoporosis is not only a women's disease. Men's bones can thin as they age just as women's do, although the disease isn't as common in men because they usually start out their adult life with much thicker bones than women. Bone thickness is different for men than women because after puberty, men have ten times as much total testosterone as women.

The most potent bone stimulator is the hormone testosterone. Testosterone provides men with very thick bones before they begin to age, so they start out ahead of women and usually stay there if they have adequate testosterone. Women go through a complete loss of estradiol and testosterone at midlife that men never experience. Men never go into true male menopause because they continue make *some* testosterone until the day they die, and that usually prevents osteoporosis.

However, some men develop osteoporosis with TDS—usually men who are genetically predisposed to having very thin bones, men who have high levels of cortisol due to severe stress or who are given cortisol-like drugs (prednisone, Medrol®) that are prescribed for asthma and autoimmune diseases, and men who lose their testosterone early in life. When TDS begins, bone thickness decreases, like it does in women after menopause. And high-risk men become osteoporotic over time.

This disease of aging can be prevented in men by replacing testosterone and increasing it to its young, healthy blood level.

Eighty-year-old Tony was short (5 feet 3 inches) for a man, and he'd suffered from severe osteoporosis since his late sixties. He was a forty-pack-per-year smoker who'd quit at age fifty-four due to worsening asthma. He'd been on steroids throughout his lifetime for asthma.

To complicate matters, Tony started out as a very poor Italian boy from Little Italy in Manhattan, growing up after the crash of 1929. He had terrible nutrition in his early life; and during his adolescent growth spurt, he had very little fresh food or necessary nutrients. Even though he was 100 percent Italian and had dark skin and eyes, he suffered for over twenty-five years from the effects of osteoporosis. It's likely that he started life with thinner-than-average bones due to all of the above factors, as well as low growth hormone during his early years, which also impacts bone density.

His suffering was intolerable. Every step he took was painful. His knees were worn away from long-distance running, and his vertebrae were damaged, which left him even shorter than before. He had used a walker and, finally, was in a wheelchair.

Never once was he treated with hormones or drugs for osteoporosis. Doctors usually think of osteoporosis as a woman's disease or consider it a normal part of aging in men, so they rarely treat men who have osteoporosis. Tony spent 25 percent of his ninety-three years in a miserable state: falling down, unable to walk, and unable to care for himself. I wouldn't wish this on anyone.

Tony was my father, and his suffering is one of the reasons I'm so dedicated to treating men with testosterone. It was a torture to watch him try to get through life as he suffered with this disease.

❏ Autoimmune Diseases: Rheumatoid Arthritis, Systemic Lupus, Crohn's Disease, Multiple Sclerosis, Scleroderma, Psoriasis, and Fibromyalgia

The risk for all adult autoimmune diseases increases as people age. That risk parallels the decrease in testosterone levels in both men and women. The onset of these diseases in women is highest after age forty and in men after age fifty, the same time when both sexes become symptomatic from testosterone deficiency.

Autoimmune diseases are, at the most basic level, an over-reaction of the immune system that causes unnecessary inflammation throughout the body. Again, we find inflammation associated with the diseases of aging. Each of these autoimmune diseases targets a different area of the body—such as the joints, the kidneys, the colon, the skin, the muscles, or the nervous tissue—and they slowly destroy otherwise healthy tissue.

All autoimmune diseases have one thing in common: they are essentially the result of "friendly fire" from the immune system that's aimed at healthy, rather than sick, tissues. It begins by immunologic confusion that aims T killer cells and B white cells toward normal tissue when invaders like bacteria and viruses have stimulated the white blood cells into action. Sadly, an immune system that targets healthy tissue is hard to reprogram, and the result is a chronic illness that continues for years, causing pain and disability.

We don't know the exact trigger for each of these diseases, but viruses and exposure to chemicals have been suggested, although not yet proven. These diseases most certainly involve genetic risk, and those men with a specific genotype are at risk for developing them, but they don't occur in everyone who carries the genetic risk. There is hope for prevention by adjusting hormones and lifestyles.

Multiple sclerosis (MS) and rheumatoid arthritis (RA) are two autoimmune diseases that can occur in aging men as their testosterone becomes deficient. Jim, a friend of mine for many years, came to see me as a patient. He confided that he'd just been diagnosed with these two autoimmune diseases, and he'd had his first medical visit with two specialists. He was worried about the treatments for autoimmune diseases that suppress the immune system and the risk of cancer and death that these specialists discussed with him. I asked if I could look at his blood work before he started on immune-suppressant drugs. Jim agreed, and I found that he had very low total T and free T.

I offered Jim testosterone pellets as an alternative to the dangerous medications that were recommended by his specialists. Of course, he could always choose to go back to those doctors if the testosterone didn't work. We inserted his pellets and within two months, his blood tests had normalized, and he had no symptoms of MS or RA.

Jim went back to his specialists one more time. One of them was ecstatic and asked to meet me; the other was angry and disparaged me. Jim simply smiled because he was better, and his life was back on track. Two years later there was no sign of either disease, and he is still disease free!

Everything that activates the immune system can result in an autoimmune disease under the right circumstances. Here's a list of things that can suppress and confuse a guy's immune system, leading to autoimmune disease.

Triggers and Factors That Cause Autoimmune Diseases:
- Aging
- Loss of testosterone
- Viral infections
- Cancer drugs
- Low cortisol
- Bacterial and yeast-like infection

All these factors, either by themselves or combined, can cause a man with a genetic predisposition to have an overreaction of the immune system and cause an autoimmune response that results in lifelong disease.

If you have relatives with an autoimmune disease, then you may be at risk for developing one of them after you have a viral or bacterial infection. Of course, the best prevention is not to get sick; however, that's not realistic. The best thing at-risk patients can do to prevent autoimmune diseases is to regularly replace lost testosterone with pellets.

> **The best way to prevent autoimmune diseases is not to get sick; however, that's not realistic. The best thing at-risk patients can do is to regularly replace lost testosterone with pellets.**

You may have heard commercials on golf programs that advertise prescription medication to treat the autoimmune disease psoriatic arthritis. A certain golf celebrity has become the "poster child" for a drug that suppresses the immune system and decreases the self-destruction of the healthy tissue by an autoimmune disease. Although the product does decrease the symptoms and pain, it also shuts down the *normal* defenses the body needs to prevent viral infections, fungal infections, bacterial infections, and even cancer.

These biologics are not the only treatment available, and they should be used only as a last-ditch effort. There's a safer answer. I've seen what the natural treatment of testosterone can do for many autoimmune diseases. The results are remarkable, and the research is present in medical literature but is buried in the endocrine journals. Endocrinologists typically don't treat these autoimmune disorders. Any man with an adult autoimmune disease should add testosterone pellets to his treatment regimen.

❏ Dementia and Alzheimer's Disease

Most Americans know that if you live long enough, your body, brain, or both will malfunction. The aging human body is like a car with 250,000 miles on the odometer; we won't last forever. And that is true of the brain, as well as the rest of the body. The loss of thinking, problem-solving, and language are what strikes fear in most adult hearts. This fear is compounded if you've watched your parents lose their ability to recognize family members and communicate. To make it worse, the mysterious disease we call Alzheimer's disease is often familial, so when we care for our parents, we may be seeing what our own future holds in a few decades.

What if there were one treatment you could take today that would delay this living death sentence, this source of fear and anxiety? The good news is that there is, and I want everyone to know that there's hope that you won't have to experience what your parents lived through.

> **What if there were one treatment you could take today that would delay this living death sentence, this source of fear and anxiety?**

Before we talk about how to avoid dementia and Alzheimer's disease, I need to lay a little groundwork about dementia, which is the umbrella term that covers many conditions that are defined as including cognitive defects (or in simpler terms, the inability to think) as their primary symptom.

Dementia affects 35.6 million people worldwide, and the number is increasing each year. There are many types of dementia, and Alzheimer's disease is *just one* of many that's included in this group of degenerative brain diseases.

It's ironic that the more successful we are at staying alive, the more often we suffer from degenerative diseases that strip us of our humanity.

The Nature and Causes of Dementia

Symptoms of dementia often begin when a man loses his ability to remember people's names or recall the term for certain items. That's usually followed by an inability to remember recent events, which then progresses to an inability to remember events from the more distant past. We all have some of these symptoms a few times a day or week without actually having dementia, and we associate more frequent incidents of poor recall with aging. However, when the symptoms progress and worsen, an evaluation to rule out one of the dementias is warranted.

Many things can trigger dementia. Strokes, which are caused by vascular clots or leakage, are one of the most common culprits because they damage large areas in the brain. It's like being hit with a "smart bomb" that wipes out an area of the brain from a leak in a blood vessel or a blood clot that robs the area of oxygen. This is more common as we age because aging, and all that comes with it, causes blood vessels to narrow and weaken. And blood vessels become more susceptible to rupture when exposed to high blood pressure, which increases with age.

Both arterial blockage and vascular rupture can cause the permanent death of parts of the brain. When this brain damage affects areas dedicated to thought or memory, it's called "vascular dementia." When we're young, we can regenerate some of the brain that was damaged; but as we get older and are under the influence of low testosterone and low growth hormone levels, we don't heal as well and the damage becomes permanent.

Alzheimer's disease is a different physiologic process from vascular dementia. Alzheimer's disease is a genetic disease that can be tested for with a simple blood test called ApoE test. Normal patients have test results of Apo E2/E2 or Apo E2/E3. Moderately at-risk people show results of Apo E3/3 or Apo E3/4. If the diagnostic genetic test result is Apo E4/E4, the person is at high risk for getting the disease as they age. Many people who have Alzheimer's disease in their family don't want to take the test for fear of the results.

Alzheimer's is fundamentally a process that deposits material like rust on the neurons of the brain. The rust piles up and short-circuits the thought process and literally kills the neurons. The massive number of neuron deaths progressively make the brain shrink. The "rust" is really a substance called "amyloid" coating the neurons, combined with inflammation. The normal brain cells can't replenish the number of dying ones, so a man slowly loses his memory and even his thoughts.

Dementia can also be caused by traumatic head injury, like concussions suffered during competitive contact sports or from a single incident such as an auto accident. In these situations, dementia may not show up immediately because the real injury is often to the pituitary gland, which struggles to work effectively for a period of time before malfunctioning. When injured, the pituitary either stops or decreases secreting growth hormone or stimulating testosterone, thyroid, and adrenals. The onset of dementia can be delayed for twenty or more years, eventually accelerating the aging impact on the brain. The brain fails to repair itself because of lack of anabolic hormones, and thus shrinks. The outcome is loss of effective memory and problem-solving ability and, over time, dementia.

Athletes who've experienced head injuries and auto-accident victims represent a relatively new area of study for endocrinologists and neurologists. The National Football League has become increasingly aware of the potential long-term effects of repetitive concussion. The current expert on this subject is Dr. Mark Gordon, medical director of Millennium Health Centers in Southern California, who has just released a book for doctors called *The Clinical Application of Interventional Endocrinology.* It features a chapter on the outcome of head injury in athletics and includes a discussion of how hormone replacement can reverse the hormonal deficits caused by trauma.

But there is hope that we can prevent this scenario! Please read on for the preventive treatment recommendations.

How to Prevent Dementia

Good nutrition, decreased inflammation, normal cholesterol, normal blood pressure, normal body weight, and daily exercise all help prevent strokes and the other changes associated with brain aging. The most important factor in preventing stroke and the damages of aging, however, may be the replacement of all hormones that decrease with age: testosterone, growth hormone, thyroid, insulin, and corticosteroids. Without the replacement of the most important brain regenerative hormone—testosterone—our brains are more sensitive to the effects of low oxygen and are more likely to be lined with cholesterol plaque. They don't have the anabolic effect of testosterone that heals them. This is one of the reasons dementia is the likely outcome of stroke in older patients.

How Does Testosterone Prevent the Onset and Progression of Dementia?

Testosterone prevents dementia through several mechanisms: it repairs neurons in the brain and prevents their death; it increases production of neurotransmitters, even when they are stressed; it decreases inflammation; it decreases shrinkage of the brain after andropause with aging; and it increases blood flow and oxygen to the brain by dilating blood vessels.

Specifically, if a man's testosterone level does not remain in the young, healthy range as he ages, his brain begins to shrink and his neurons die and don't replace themselves as they age. When the process devolves to a certain point, adding testosterone can't reverse the damage.

Dementia is a quality-of-life issue, as well as a practical problem for families. This disease of aging is the most obvious motivator I can think of for replacing testosterone. It's an effective new preventive treatment for any man who wants to age with his brain intact and retain his independence.

How Soon Should I Replace Testosterone?

Timing is everything when it comes to replacing testosterone. There's a ten-year window after T declines below the young, healthy level during which you can replace T and maintain your brain size and function. T replacement delays the onset of all types of dementia by up to ten years.

The optimum time for T replacement is when symptoms of TDS *begin*, which marks the beginning of the ten-year window after which brain cells are irretrievable. Sometimes, however, we try to stop or slow the process with testosterone pellets, even for men who are beyond the ten-year window.

Alzheimer's disease increases with life expectancy unless we intervene with healthier lifestyles and testosterone replacement.

Timing is everything when it comes to replacing testosterone. There's a ten-year window after T declines to below the young, healthy level during which you can replace T and maintain your brain size and function.

In the magazine *The Australian*, Lee Dayton in his article "Experiments Pay Off in Alzheimer's Breakthrough" writes about the success of T replacement in decreasing the incidence of Alzheimer's disease in aging men and women. Testosterone decreases the pituitary hormones LH and FSH, both of which play a part in Alzheimer's disease plaque formation. If we can give enough T to decrease LH and FSH, the article suggests, we can suppress plaque formation and delay the onset of Alzheimer's disease.

A 2002 article in the *Journal of the American Medical Association* also proved that some serious cognitive diseases can be *delayed* through the use of testosterone therapy. There is sufficient scientific evidence that replacement of estradiol in women and testosterone in both sexes *prevents* dementia and Alzheimer's disease, but there is currently no evidence that replacement can *reverse or halt* the progression of the disease. And yet, other studies demonstrate that testosterone replacement can stop progression of dementia.

Reversing the Decline in Brain Power

A recent study reported on in *Endocrine News* demonstrated that replacement of testosterone that converts into dihydrotestosterone (DHT) restores not only neurotransmitters, but also the synapses and brain cells in mice. That's a whole different level of restoration! Testosterone must be replaced to defend against Alzheimer's disease. As of today, it's the only preventive method we know of.

Are there specific guidelines to make this work for you? Yes! *First, you must replace testosterone in a non-oral form.* The subcutaneously inserted testosterone pellets cross the blood-brain barrier and increase neurotransmitters better than any other form of bioidentical testosterone. Communication among neurons is quickly reestablished. Second, *you must not wait more than ten years after TDS begins to replace your testosterone.*

A word about side effects. No adverse side effects have been identified in any research we've studied related to preventing Alzheimer's disease with testosterone replacement.

Scientists worldwide are currently focusing on the explosion of Alzheimer's disease diagnosis in the aging population. Quality of life concerns as we age demand a greater focus on testosterone replacement. The encouraging results from new research indicates that if we cannot avoid Alzheimer's disease in our future, we can at least delay it by acting early!

The encouraging results indicate that if we cannot avoid Alzheimer's disease in our future, we can at least delay it by acting early!

❏ **Male Breast Cancer**

Breast cancer is much less common in men than in women, but it does occur and should be evaluated by your primary care doctor during annual checkups. Men who are at greatest risk are those who have breast cancer in their family, especially in male relatives.

The highest risk is in men born in Sicily or whose genetics are from Sicily and southern Italy. The abnormality is a genetic defect called *aromatase enzyme defect*, which drastically increases the amount of estradiol and estrone a man's testosterone produces. In Sicilian men, the breast cells have abnormal receptors and are very sensitive to estrone. When this genetic defect was discovered, a drug in a class of drugs called aromatase inhibitors (Arimidex®), which is now used for female and male breast cancer, was developed.

We currently don't have an affordable genetic test to look for the aromatase enzyme defect. But when we check men for total T, free T, estrone, and estradiol levels, we find that those with low free T, high estrone, and high estradiol possess this gene defect. Low free T decreases the body's immunity, and high estrone and estradiol stimulate man boobs and increase the risk of male breast cancer.

We treat men who have this profile with T pellets and Arimidex® to decrease the estrone and estradiol levels and to increase free testosterone. This also has the happy side effect of curing man boobs.

If a man finds a breast lump, he should see his doctor immediately for an exam, a breast ultrasound, and/or a mammogram to evaluate whether he needs a biopsy. This is a treatable disease, and a man shouldn't be embarrassed to discuss it with his doctor. We doctors have heard everything, and we're in practice to help. If the first doctor doesn't listen, then consult a breast surgeon.

❏ Cancer

All cancers are really diseases of the immune system. The primary problem isn't that the organ system has cancer; the problem is that the immune system has malfunctioned and allowed cancer cells to slip through the surveillance system. Every day, each of us makes abnormal cells that *could* become cancer, but our healthy immune systems kill those abnormal cells.

Our immune system is our "army" that protects us. The white blood cells, called T-killer cells and T-helper cells, come from the bone marrow and the thymus gland (behind the breast bone). They're the infantry that shoots down abnormal cells all day and night.

Testosterone protects us from cancer by stimulating the immune cells to do a better job of finding and killing abnormal cancers cells.

Testosterone protects us from cancer by stimulating the immune cells to do a better job of finding and killing abnormal cancer cells. When we're young, our testosterone levels are high, and we have a big thymus with lots of active "soldiers" (T-cells) that kill cancer cells. As testosterone decreases with age, the thymus shrinks, and the number and activity of the T-cells decreases. Our immune system lets its guard down, which increases our risk of getting cancer.

Factors That Increase the Risk of Cancer in Men:

- Obesity
- Genetic risk for cancer = family history of cancer
- Stress, which increases cortisol levels and suppresses the immune cells
- Heavy metals and chemicals, which increase breakage of DNA and create more precancerous cells
- Smoking, which suppresses the activity of immune cells
- Alcohol, which by stimulating the liver, prevents it from doing its job of destroying other poisons that cause cancer
- Medications that suppress immunity (autoimmune-disease drugs and steriods, for example)

If you want to decrease your risk of cancer, then clean up your act! Stop smoking, don't drink in excess, lose weight, and detox. And de-stress in natural ways: get a punching bag! And when your testosterone deficiency first becomes symptomatic, replace your testosterone with testosterone pellets.

If you want to decrease your risk of cancer, then clean up your act!

❑ Sarcopenia

Sarcopenia is the medical term for frailty. We associate aging with becoming frail. We lose muscle and fat, skin hangs off our bones, we develop stooped posture from thin bones, our gait slows, and we have less animation in our facial muscles and speech. It's excruciatingly painful to have sarcopenia and to watch it progress.

In the medical world, sarcopenia is considered an inevitable and untreatable chronic condition that occurs for years before death. In my world of preventive medicine and lifelong testosterone replacement, this condition can be avoided and treated before it becomes severe. We really don't have to become frail and rickety before we die!

We can't stop the clock, but we can replace hormones.

How and when does this condition occur? It is different for each of us, but it usually happens somewhere after seventy-five years if a man hasn't replaced his testosterone and/or growth hormone. Testosterone and growth hormone support the growth and replenishment of bones, muscle, skin, nerves, brain, and hair. Sarcopenia isn't only from aging but is also from the loss of all anabolic hormones that come from aging. We can't stop the clock, but we can replace hormones.

My dad lived to be ninety-three. He was a short but well-muscled man who worked out every day and took a handful of vitamins daily. He took good care of himself, yet at age eighty-five, he began to shrink. He lost height, his legs became bowed, and he even lost a shoe size. It was like someone had put him in the dryer for too long!

A few years after this change began, I suggested he get his testosterone level checked. He complained but finally agreed. Unfortunately, he got his lab sheet before I saw it, and he called me to proudly tell me his total T level was normal! I knew that couldn't be true because of how he looked, so I asked for the specific numbers.

He told me his total T level was 8 ng/dl, and the lab sheet said "normal." Normal total T is 400-1,500 ng/dl for any age. We compare the levels of T to young, healthy males twenty to forty years old, just like we compare bones of males of any age to twenty-nine-year-old males. There's no known normal for eighty-five-year-old men, so the lab just put in a low number. I'm still flabbergasted that they would do this! Because the lab had never tracked "normal" or average for this age group, they just made it up!

That was it for my dad. His doctor didn't listen to me, and he trusted his doctor, so I lost the battle and spent the next eight years taking care of him as he shriveled away, body and soul. If I could have put him on T pellets, I believe he would have lived longer and independently, instead of being relegated to an assisted-living facility in a wheelchair.

❏ Risk of Early Mortality

It's been proven over and over that testosterone decreases both the incidence and severity of all the diseases of aging that eventually result in fatal complications and death. One by one, medical articles are being published in respected medical journals that plainly state that replacing testosterone, or normalizing testosterone levels to optimal levels, decreases illnesses that lead to death! Indeed, every month, *The Journal of Endocrinology and Metabolism* contains numerous articles that justify the use of testosterone to keep aging men healthy and disease-free; yet mainstream medicine refuses to advocate the use of testosterone to treat and prevent the diseases of aging!

Why haven't you heard of this? I don't think that there's some evil plot to emasculate men as they age or to cause men to die early. But in view of all the medical studies that have concluded that replacing testosterone is the safest way to preserve health, improve quality of life, and even extend life, I can't understand why medical gurus don't make it mandatory to offer testosterone in its safest forms to men over age fifty.

CHAPTER 4

Testosterone Pellets: The Best Option for Men

When you reach the age when your body no longer makes the hormones that kept you sexually active and healthy, it's time to choose the testosterone replacement that will work best for your needs. Most men think of testosterone replacement the same way they've been taught to approach all medications—as one size fits all. However, testosterone replacement isn't like that. In fact, it's a lot like buying a car. There are a number of models to choose from, and the differences are profound.

Perhaps you look for certain things when purchasing a car: quality, comfort, reliability, and value. I suggest you do the same when shopping for testosterone replacement. Here are some valid questions to ask:

- What type of testosterone is the *easiest to use* with the *least upkeep*? In other words, which type must be dosed the fewest times per day, week, or year?

- Which testosterone provides the *best quality?*

- What kind of testosterone has the *fewest problems* (side effects)?

- Which one will *last the longest?*

- Which testosterone is the *best value for my money?*
- Which testosterone *"rides the smoothest"?*

The problem with T is that there's no *Consumer Reports* where you can compare and contrast your testosterone choices and make an informed selection. In this arena, the only information available is found in pharmaceutical commercials, advice from doctors who are informed (bought) by drug companies, or on the internet. It isn't easy to compare testosterone preparations, so I'm offering you the results of my research that led me to exclusively prescribe and use *testosterone pellets* for my male patients.

It isn't easy to compare testosterone preparations, so I'm offering you the results of my research that led me to exclusively prescribe and use *testosterone pellets* for my male patients.

How Do the Ease of Treatment and the Cost of Different Forms of Testosterone Compare?

There are many types of testosterone and each "feels" different to the man who is taking it. That's why it's necessary to compare the different forms to determine the best possible outcome in terms of how you feel, the most convenient delivery system, and which form fits your budget and is the safest for you.

When comparing different forms of testosterone ask:

- What's it made of? (natural vegetable source or chemical invention?)
- What is the delivery method? (oral pill, gel to rub on the skin, wearable patch, muscle injection, subcutaneous injection, or pellet inserted in fat tissue?)
- How often must you remember to take it?

- What's the cost? (important to know since testosterone in any form is rarely covered by insurance)

In the table on the next page, I've divided the forms of T replacement into groups based on how they're administered, because the way the testosterone is given usually determines how often it's taken and its overall effectiveness.

Every man will have his own criteria regarding what's most important to him. Some men will want the easiest and most convenient method of testosterone delivery, so they don't have to think about taking it every day. For these men, pellets inserted into the fat of their hip or flank once every six months will help them absorb all the testosterone they've been prescribed without constantly dosing themselves.

Other men may want to have full control over their testosterone doses, which means dosing themselves—even if they have to do it twice per day, every day! Still others will want the form that costs the least. The least-expensive choice is to take testosterone cypionate intramuscular injections, but that requires you to visit your doctor every two weeks to get the shot.

Consider the table on the next page. Low cost means more time and effort.

Overall, bioidentical pellets are the easiest form of testosterone replacement for men. They require a man to think about his testosterone only twice a year when he goes to the doctor's office to have his pellets inserted. This dosing schedule doesn't conflict with travel and doesn't involve transporting drugs with you when you travel to other countries. In addition, you don't have to go to the pharmacy every month for a prescription or visit your doctor every one or two weeks to get an injection.

Over the years, I've learned that if a treatment isn't easy to follow, patients will simply give it up. T replacement is for life, and it must be delivered on a consistent basis because it's vital to your productivity and sexuality. By making it easy to take in bioidentical pellet form, our preferred testosterone treatment allows us to give you a consistent, accurate dose, as well as ensure compliance. With pellets, you won't forget your testosterone.

Comparison of Different Testosterone Delivery Systems In Terms of Ease of Treatment and Cost

This table compares the ease of taking each form of testosterone, which is what determines whether you'll follow through and stay on that form of testosterone.

Easiest = ✔   Hardest = ✔✔✔✔

Also compared is the overall cost of treatment, which includes what you spend at a pharmacy and at a doctor's office.

Least Expensive = $ Most Expensive = $$$$$$

	Bioidentical T Pellets	Transdermal (Patch & Gel)	Oral T = Pill	T Lozenge	T Cypionate Injection
Ease of Use	✔	✔✔✔✔✔	✔✔	✔✔✔✔	✔✔✔✔✔
Brand Names	None, Pure T, Bioidentical	Androgel®, Androderm® Patch	Testosterone Unadecanoate	None, Bioidentical	None, Generic
Where Administered	Doctor's Office	Home	Home	Home	Doctor's Office
Times You Must Remember to Dose	Twice a Year	1-2 Times a Day	Weekly	1-2 Times a Day	Weekly
Insurance Coverage	No	Rare	No	No	Sometimes
Annual Doctor Visits	2	2-6	4	2-4	24
Cost	$$$$	$$$$$	$$	$$$$	$$$

If you're someone who can't remember to take your vitamins, then you won't remember to take your testosterone in the form of gels, patches, or lozenges either! If you travel for work or play or live in two or three different places (summer and winter houses), then getting pellets two times a year will be the most efficient and convenient form of T replacement. If cost is a more important factor for you than the time spent to get your T replacement, then sitting in a doctor's office every two weeks to get your shot might be the best choice for you.

There's been a lot of research on patients who are required to take their medications daily or even twice daily. Most of the study patients forgot their meds two times per week. If a man has to dose his own testosterone two times per day, it's unlikely that he'll ever take the second dose! If daily dosing of T is this ineffective, it means that the treatment won't be successful. The purpose of treating men with testosterone is to alleviate their symptoms and prevent the diseases of aging. Neither of these goals can be attained if the testosterone prescribed isn't taken.

Because I'm concerned about my patients' health, I offer only testosterone pellets. Testosterone pellets treat the most symptoms of TDS in the safest way, at moderate price, with the fewest risks. Further, when using pellets, I don't have to worry if the man is actually getting his testosterone dose or of if he's taking twice the amount I ordered by dosing it himself at home with a gel or lozenge. I administer the pellet dose, and I know exactly what he's receiving.

With T pellets, you simply "get your testosterone and forget it!" two times per year. You comply with the recommended dosage without additional worry, cost, or time-consuming strategies. Pellets are your best choice for lifelong testosterone replacement.

How Do the Medical Benefits and Risks of Different Forms of Testosterone Compare?

The most important factor when choosing a form of T replacement (after whether you'll actually take it), is to pick the one with the greatest benefit and least risk. It's difficult to compare how youthful each form of testosterone might make a man feel, and I won't even attempt to do that. But I can tell you that pellets *do* make my patients feel young again, and they tell me that *that* feeling is one they've never received from any other form of testosterone.

The table on the next page compares the benefits of the different forms of testosterone replacement.

Comparison of the Benefits of Different Forms of Testosterone Replacement

Most Beneficial= ★★★★★   Least Beneficial= ★

Benefits of T Replacement ↓	Bioidentical T Pellets	Transdermal (Patch & Gel)	Oral T = Pill	T Lozenge	T Cypionate Shot
Treats Ed	★★★★★	★	★★★★	★	★★★★★
↑ Mood	★★★★★	★	★★	★★	★★★★
↓ Cardiac Risk	★★★★★	★	★	★★★	★
↑ Muscle Mass	★★★★★	★	★★★	★★	★★★★★
Weight Loss	★★★★★	★	★★★	★★	★★★★
↑ Sex Drive	★★★★★	★	★★★★	★	★★★★★
↓ Ldl Cholesterol	★★★★★	★★	★	★★	★
↓ Estrogen	★★★★★	★	★	★★	★★★

This comparison is based on my clinical experience with my medical practice and a review of published medical research.

I recommend that you not only look at the benefits of your T-replacement options but also consider the risks. Some of these risks may mean very little to a man whose only problem is low T, but they'll mean more to a man who has liver disease or diabetes, or who has had a heart attack.

In general, T pellets have fewer risks than any other form of testosterone replacement, which means a healthier life for you and fewer worries for your doctor. Take a look at the table on the next page to see if any of the risks listed might interfere with any medical problems you have. If you aren't sure, then put the item on a list of things to talk to your doctor about when you have your initial consultation.

Comparison of the Risks of Different Forms of Testosterone Replacement

Lowest Risk= ✖   Greatest Risk= ✖✖✖✖✖

Risks of T Replacement ↓	Bioidentical T Pellets	Transdermal (Patch & Gel)	Oral T = Pill	T Lozenge	T Cypionate Injection
Infertility	✖	✖	✖✖✖	✖	✖✖✖✖✖
Liver Damage	✖	✖	✖✖✖✖✖	✖	✖
Man Boobs	✖	✖✖✖✖✖	✖✖✖✖✖	✖✖✖	✖✖
↑ Belly Fat	✖	✖✖✖✖	✖✖✖	✖✖✖	✖✖
Hair Loss	✖	✖	✖✖✖	✖	✖✖✖✖✖
Blood Clots	✖	✖✖	✖✖✖✖	✖✖	✖✖
Enlarged Prostate	✖✖ first 2 months, then ✖	✖✖	✖✖✖✖	✖✖	✖✖✖
Erythrocytosis	✖✖✖	✖	✖✖✖	✖	✖✖✖✖

The comparison in this table is based on my clinical experience in my medical practice and a review of published medical research. The lowest-risk, most-effective type of testosterone replacement is clearly bioidentical testosterone pellets.

Testosterone Gel: The Most Common Testosterone Replacement

Let's say you arrive at your first testosterone replacement therapy session with the complaint, "I have no sex drive" or "I'm tired." That's when most doctors pull out their pad and write a prescription for what the latest drug rep gave them samples of: testosterone gel. Easy for the doctor, but not so easy for you. In fact, using a gel is such a constant bother that it's the rare man who actually complies with the directions and applies it twice a day. And even if they do, there's no guarantee they'll get better.

What usually happens is this: You apply the gel under your arms twice a day for two weeks. You start to feel better for the first month but then forget to use it, or you get busy and your symptoms return. So you call your doctor, who doubles the dose. Again, you're better for a month or so, perhaps less, and then it's back to square one because *you just can't remember to apply the gel or be bothered with the mess during your work day.* You either get frustrated and quit, or you continue the same pattern until you're using eight times the daily recommended dose and feel worse for it. By this time, you may have grown voluptuous breasts and gained ten pounds of belly fat, and your thyroid may have crashed! Needless to say, you're more miserable than ever.

Why does this happen? The FDA and pharmaceutical companies that produce gel testosterone are well aware of the problem. It happens because more than half of the testosterone in prescription testosterone gel is converted into estrogens as it's absorbed through the skin! Remember how T can convert into estrone and estradiol? When gels convert into estrogen, it can cause a large amount of SHBG (sex hormone binding globulin) that binds up the *active* testosterone and leaves men with *very little free T as well as elevated estrogens.*

You feel better at first because you're absorbing 40 percent of the testosterone as *testosterone* and 60 percent as *estrogen*. But over the following months, more and more T becomes estrogen, and soon your active testosterone is bound up. So you go back to the doctor to complain about your symptoms. The doctor doesn't know what's really happening—not because he's incompetent but because this is a minor part of his practice—so he does the logical thing, which is to increase the dose.

What the doctor doesn't know is that *the more T gel you take, the more estrogen is produced. And more estrogen lowers free T.* To restore your libido and make you healthy, you must have >129 ng/ml of free T. When T gel becomes estrogen and free T becomes low again, you've wasted your time and money, not to mention the sloppy inconvenience of applying the gel, and your free T never even gets to 129 ng/ml. The sad part is that your physician may not even know why your treatment isn't working.

That's why I never prescribe transdermal gel to men.

Potential Side Effects of Testosterone Replacement

Erythrocytosis (Too Many Red Blood Cells)

Erythrocytosis is a genetic vulnerability that is made worse by high T levels. It is defined as having a high level of hemoglobin and a hematocrit over 50 percent. The primary problem with erythrocytosis is that "thick" blood that is hard to pump puts stress on the heart. Testosterone replacement makes this worse because T increases iron absorption, which thickens blood.

The only *symptom* of erythrocytosis is high blood pressure and a red face. "Thick" blood caused by erythrocytosis causes the heart to work harder and impairs the free flow of blood in the vessels. This can eventually cause heart disease, heart failure, or both. It is easily treated with regular blood donation.

Hemochromatosis (Too Much Stored Iron)

Hemochromatosis is another genetic problem that causes excess iron to deposit in healthy organs, where it acts as a heavy metal and damages the organs in which it collects. Hemochromatosis can deposit iron in the liver, testes, brain, eye, pituitary—anywhere. If it's undiagnosed and untreated, it can cause liver failure, blindness, psychiatric disorders, and testicular failure. T makes hemochromatosis worse.

A man can be asymptomatic or he may feel tired and sick—until he's treated with phlebotomies or blood donation. These two conditions are worsened by testosterone replacement of any kind because testosterone increases iron absorption and makes more red blood cells.

Conversion into Estrogens

All men make increasing amounts of estrogen from their testosterone as they age. Excess estrogen is a problem for men that causes several side effects and medical problems. The desirable treatment goal is to treat this by lowering estrogens, not to wipe out all estrogen in a man's system because that's not healthy. The tricky part is to strike a balance and maintain a small amount of estrogen without getting too much.

The natural aging process causes ever-increasing estradiol and estrone levels, which lead to belly fat, male breast development, prostate enlargement, blood clot formation, and imbalanced emotions. Because many testosterone preparations almost completely convert into estrone and estradiol, they add to the naturally occurring testosterone decline and estrogen increase in aging men—and they obliterate the benefits of testosterone replacement. The first step to avoid these side effects is to select a testosterone preparation that does not create extra estrogen. Such is the benefit of bioidentical testosterone pellets.

A certain percentage of men convert testosterone into estrogen prematurely, beginning in their early forties. These men are generally plagued by a genetic defect in their aromatase enzyme (the enzyme that converts T into estrogen). As we have noted, their genetic lineage is usually from Italy and Sicily or Southern Europe.

The remedy to manage this issue in all aging men—and particularly those who have this enzyme defect—is to choose a low estrogen-converting kind of testosterone and to prescribe Arimidex® so the testosterone doesn't turn into estrogen!

Elevated Dihydrotestosterone

Testosterone replacement can be complicated by elevated dihydrotestosterone (DHT), which is a normal by-product of testosterone. But when there's too much of it, it can cause benign prostatic hyperplasia (prostate gland enlargement), male-pattern baldness, elevated LDL cholesterol, acne, hyperhidrosis (extreme and excessive sweating), and superabundant body hair. It would be easy to wipe out DHT production, but that would be a mistake because it's necessary for sex drive, sexual response, muscle mass development, and brain neurotransmitters that create energy and sexuality. Our goal is to keep DHT in balance without totally suppressing it.

I treat elevated DHT that's accompanied by the symptoms above with saw palmetto, an herb that blocks the production of DHT from testosterone. This herb is found in most over-the-counter prostate formulas and is produced in a strength that doesn't decrease the production of DHT below an optimum level.

If saw palmetto isn't strong enough, I prescribe a very low dose of finasteride, used every other day to every third day to control the production of DHT. With testosterone pellets, I rarely need finasteride to prevent the side effects that are secondary to an elevated DHT. If the drug is necessary, it works quickly to shrink the prostate, so this therapy is not always necessary long term.

Unfounded Concern About Prostate Cancer and Testosterone

The most prevalent myth about testosterone replacement—any form of T replacement—is that it causes prostate cancer. This untruth has been propagated by both doctors and fear-mongering websites. Doctors repeat this false information because they learned it in medical school decades ago. This conclusion was based on a study of *only two men in the 1960s* who *already had* prostate cancer. And their cancer was exacerbated when exposed to testosterone. Only one man remained in the study, plus the research was not peer-reviewed or conducted as a double-blind study—the standard for current accepted research.

But it's what I was taught in medical school in the late seventies. My question then is the same as it is now: *If testosterone stimulates prostate cells to become cancerous, then why do young men with very high T have an absence of prostate cancer, and aging men with low T levels have a high rate of prostate cancer?* It still doesn't make sense.

For decades, testosterone treatment was based on this faulty research until Abraham Morgantaler, MD, FACS, of Harvard Medical School began to study the causes of prostate cancer and the effects of testosterone on the prostate. His book *Testosterone for Life!* describes his extensive research, and he concludes that testosterone is an anti-cancer hormone that stimulates the protection of the immune system; it *does not* cause prostate cancer.

My favorite example in his study that proves that T is safe—and is even protective—is when he biopsied both old men with precancerous prostate cells and young men with normal prostate cells. He then bathed the old precancerous prostate cells with the young men's testosterone-rich blood, and the young cells with the old men's low-testerosterone blood. When bathed in the high-T blood from the young men, the old men's precancerous prostate cells became normal. The young men's cells became abnormal when grown in the low-T environment of the older men's blood!

Many other studies later, Dr. Morgantaler is now on a quest to retrain the medical community and its male patients to stop rejecting testosterone treatment as men age because of the risk of prostate cancer. It may be decades before the medical mainstream changes its collective mind regarding testosterone and prostate cancer. In the meantime, fear of a treatment that can be very effective for preventing future diseases—as well as alleviate the symptoms of aging—seems unwise, particularly when the treatment can produce such desired results.

So if increasing T levels don't cause prostate cancer in aging men, what are the factors that do? As men age and testosterone drops, they naturally make more estrogen in the form of estrone and more dihydrotestosterone (DHT), both of which increase the size of the prostate. And an enlarged prostate is a precursor to prostate cancer. Low T also decreases the effectiveness of the entire immune system, which protected them from all cancers when they were younger. As men age, improving testosterone and increasing T-killer cells and T-helper cells decreases the risk of cancer of every type.

The best choice of T replacement for any and all men is bioidentical testosterone pellets injected subcutaneously every six months.

That's not to say that testosterone replacement is without risks—there's a risk to any medical treatment. But there's also a risk of *not* taking a treatment to prevent or treat an illness. You must weigh both the benefits and risks of testosterone before rejecting it outright.

I've described the most direct path to a low-risk life after age fifty. The choice to replace the testosterone that kept you healthy when you were young and virile is weighed against the risks highlighted throughout this chapter. At this point, the decision is yours.

The best choice of T replacement for any and all men is bioidentical testosterone pellets injected subcutaneously every six months. If you have symptoms of low T and/or are afraid of the genetic diseases that run in your family, then all you need to do is find a doctor in your area to provide you with testosterone pellets.

CHAPTER 5

Interpreting Your Blood Tests

By now you may have determined that you have the symptoms of TDS and want to explore testosterone replacement with long-lasting bioidentical testosterone pellets.

We take the direct approach in my office, and that starts with qualifying you as a good candidate for testosterone pellet therapy. Before you come to my office for your initial visit, you'll have an appointment at the lab to get your blood drawn. Then I'll review both your complete medical history and the results of the comprehensive panel of specific blood tests before we meet.

If this approach seems unusual, it is; however, it's the most economical and efficient way to treat men with testosterone. Usually, your insurance will pay for your lab tests, and you'll only have to invest about twenty minutes of your time to fill out a medical history form online before you ever take your wallet out. Because we qualify candidates up front, the men I can't help aren't burdened by coming to the office and being disappointed. This process also weeds out young men who make appointments for testosterone treatments for body building that they don't need.

> **All hormones in a man's body must be normalized and his habits adjusted to bring him back to health, which is why the blood tests are critical.**

During my review of your medical information, I spend about an hour going over your chart and hormone levels to develop a specific treatment plan before you ever come to see me. It's much more expedient for you because we start treating you at your first visit, so you'll feel better within a month.

I'm not like some other doctors who pass out testosterone like it's candy, and I don't want to be included in that group of physicians. My goal for every man is to replace *all* hormones—not just testosterone—that have become deficient due to age or injury and to restore him back to a young, healthy blood level *for a man between twenty and forty years old*. All hormones in a man's body must be normalized and his habits adjusted to bring him back to health, which is why the blood tests are critical.

This chapter contains a list of the tests I order before the first treatment. You'll notice an asterisk by the blood tests that we repeat four to five months later, which show how you metabolize your testosterone. If you're evaluated by a doctor who doesn't explain your blood work to you—or if you forget what she or he said—then use this chapter as a reference to understand each standard and nonstandard test that we order.

> **Losing your testosterone is the beginning of the end. Just like falling dominos, the first markers of illness and future disease begin when testosterone decreases, resulting in disease and misery for the individual, followed by a loss of strength and sexuality, and finally a shorter life span.**

Losing your testosterone is the beginning of the end. Just like falling dominos, the first markers of illness and future disease begin when testosterone decreases, resulting in disease and misery for the individual, followed by a loss of strength and sexuality, and finally a shorter life span. That doesn't have to happen to you.

Preparing for Your Blood Tests

Proper preparation for your blood tests is essential for accurate results. These are the important guidelines that you must follow:

- Your blood must be drawn before noon, preferably at 8 a.m. The significant hormones that we test for are highest in the morning, and it's easier to compare them to young, healthy normal levels at that time of day.

- You must prepare for your prostate cancer screening (PSA) test, which I draw before treatment and every year after that until you are sixty years old. *You must not have sex, exercise, ride a bike, sit in a hot tub, or have a rectal exam or an enema (yes, some people still do those) for thirty-six hours before the test.* If you violate these rules, you stand a chance of having a falsely high level of PSA. If that's the case, the test will have to be repeated, or you may be sent to a urologist for a prostate biopsy. If you're taking the drug allopurinal, stop taking it for three days before the test because it can falsely elevate your results.

- You must fast for twelve hours before your blood is drawn—no food or drink except water after 8 p.m. the night before. You can drink plenty of water, but you should not take your medications until after your blood is drawn.

Interpreting Your Blood Tests

There are some important things for you to remember as you review your test results:

- What's considered "normal" for hormones is *not* the numbers printed on the "normal range" on your lab results. Those numbers represent the average blood level *for your age*, or even the average of the tests they ran at a particular laboratory that day! When hormones decline with age and leave men ill, the average for the "ill and aging group of men who are your age" is *unhealthy*. That's not what we're aiming for.

In your pellets, I provide you with the levels you had when you were thirty-something and felt virile and energetic.

- To determine your basic health and establish baseline blood levels, I include tests that indicate medical illnesses and/or signify a high risk for future illness that might complicate testosterone pellet replacement. When we normalize your testosterone, estrone, and thyroid levels, these health tests usually improve drastically when they're repeated. There can be many consequences of hormone deficiency, and we look for those levels that indicate current illness and potential future illness, so we can quantitatively record your improvement after treatment with testosterone pellets.

- The "normals" listed in our panel for the health tests (metabolic panel, lipids, blood counts) are the levels seen in healthy men *of any age*.

- Four to five months after your first pellet insertion, we draw your blood again to chart your improvement. We compare the change in hormone levels, as well as other health markers such as blood sugar and lipid panels—all of which improve with testosterone replacement. Often our patients can go off their other drugs, like statins for high cholesterol and hypertensive medications for high blood pressure, within the first year of receiving testosterone pellets. This will not happen if you take other forms of testosterone.

Panel of Blood Tests

Listed on the next page are the blood tests that should be drawn by an experienced doctor who plans to replace your testosterone. Those with an asterisk (*) are the tests to repeat four to five months after the first pellet insertion.

Hormone Tests:

- ❏ Total testosterone*
- ❏ Free testosterone (unbound—the active form of testosterone)*
- ❏ Estrone*
- ❏ Estradiol*
- ❏ IGF-1 (growth hormone test)*
- ❏ 8 a.m. cortisol*
- ❏ LH*, FSH
- ❏ DHT (dihydroteststerone)*
- ❏ TSH*, free T3*, free T4*
- ❏ Prolactin

Cardiac Risk Tests:

- ❏ Total cholesterol, LDL cholesterol, HDL cholesterol*
- ❏ Triglycerides*
- ❏ Cardiac CRP*
- ❏ Homocysteine

Medical Health Tests:

- ❏ Metabolic panel* (liver and kidney evaluation, fasting blood sugar)
- ❏ CBC*: red blood count, white blood count, platelets
- ❏ Ferritin
- ❏ PSA (prostate cancer screening test) if you are under sixty or you are over sixty and are at high risk

These tests reveal a great deal about your health and hormonal condition, and I review the results before you come to your first appointment. The most important question we're answering is whether you can benefit from testosterone replacement.

Abnormal Blood Tests That Could Prevent You from Receiving T Pellets

When reviewing your initial blood work, I look for things that would indicate that testosterone shouldn't be prescribed, such as a high PSA count. This screening test results in a number that's over 4.0 in men with prostate cancer, and it's often high in men without prostate cancer. This would prevent me from prescribing T pellets until your urologist confirms that you don't have prostate cancer.

An extremely high red blood cell count is another contraindication to testosterone pellets until your blood level is lowered. Because testosterone increases the absorption of iron, adding more testosterone can worsen that condition by stimulating the production of more red blood cells. In such cases, we recommend the patient make a blood donation every six weeks to remove red blood cells until his level is normal.

There are also rare conditions that can be discovered in blood work that could prevent treatment, but they're found only infrequently and aren't a problem for the average man.

Explanation of and Treatment for Abnormal Blood Labs

No matter how thorough I am, I find that regular patients have a hard time absorbing all the information about their labs. There's a lot of information to retain, and much of it is rather complicated medical jargon. So I give them the information in this chapter in handouts.

If you've already had your labs drawn, you can use this section to get a general idea if you would be a candidate for testosterone replacement. Remember that different labs use different units of measure and different methods of measuring hormones. I base the lab values below on the units used by the national lab, Quest Diagnostics.

Blood Tests That Measure Men's Sex Hormones

Testosterone loss usually begins after age forty in men. Symptoms often begin around age fifty-five, but in the last decade TDS began to be evident earlier. TDS is considered to be treatable when men have symptoms at any age, as well as when their blood tests show their levels have fallen below what is normal for men between the ages of twenty and forty.

Abnormal Levels:

- ❏ Total testosterone < 400 ng/dl and free T < 129 ng/ml are inadequate testosterone levels.

If total testosterone is greater than 400 ng/dl, then a man is making an adequate amount for most men, though some men will still be symptomatic over 400 ng/dl, especially if their free T (the active form of testosterone) is less than 129 ng/ml. *Treatment: Testosterone pellets dosed to last four to six months, 10 mg per day or 1,800 mg.*

The Decrease in Active (Free) Testosterone Has a Double Impact After Age 50
The total decreases and the percentage of the total decreases

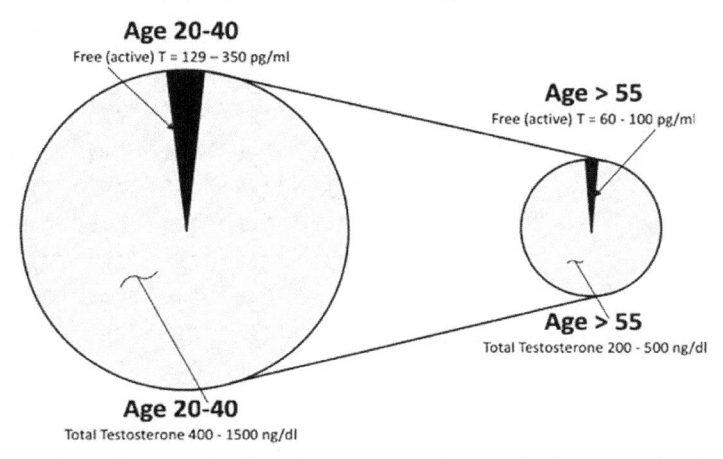

Age 20-40
Free (active) T = 129 – 350 pg/ml

Age > 55
Free (active) T = 60 - 100 pg/ml

Age > 55
Total Testosterone 200 - 500 ng/dl

Age 20-40
Total Testosterone 400 - 1500 ng/dl

As men age, the amount of total testosterone they make decreases drastically, and the percentage of active T decreases to a level that is not adequate for normalcy.

❑ Estrone (E1) (>30 pg/ml)

This is an estrogen that causes visible aging, belly fat, man boobs, and mental confusion. Too much estrone causes testosterone to be inactivated. Some men genetically make too much of this early on. In cases such as this, estrone inactivates their T even though they are making enough total T—and even if they aren't old yet. Other men drink too much alcohol and get fat, which also produces estrone.
Treatment: I treat high estrone with Arimidex® orally or in the T pellets called testosterone/anastrazole pellets. I also use a supplement called DIM (diindolylmethane) that works in a similar way to block the production of estrone.

❑ Estradiol (E2) (>40 pg/ml)

This estrogen does the same thing as E1. It's treated the same way as high estrone, too. Men need a small amount of both estradiol and estrone to keep their brain and bones healthy, so it must be managed carefully.
Treatment: Arimidex® orally or in medicated pellets and/or DIM (diindolylmethane).

❑ Low DHT (<25 ng/dl)

Dihydrotestosterone (DHT) is a by-product of testosterone and is active in hair follicles and causes hair loss; however, it also crosses the blood-brain barrier; travels into the brain; and stimulates sex drive, increases muscle mass, and produces oil in the skin. Low DHT causes a lack of the good effects of DHT, and too much causes baldness, low voice, prostate enlargement, and difficulty urinating.
Treatment: When DHT is low, replace T to young, healthy levels and treat with supplements DHEA and pregnenolone.

❑ High DHT (>79 ng/dl)

This means that your total testosterone has decreased because of two things: you produce too much DHT, and you convert usable T into too much DHT, which is a waste of your testosterone. Even though normal levels of DHT are needed for sex drive and muscle growth, excessive DHT can cause additional problems for men. Too much DHT stimulates growth of the prostate, which makes urinating difficult, and increases baldness and acne.

Treatment: Saw palmetto or finasteride given in a low dose decreases DHT and increases T levels.

Pituitary Hormone Tests: Normal and Abnormal

IGF-1 (growth hormone test), prolactin, LH, and FSH

Optimal IGF-1 (growth hormone) level at any age is (>150-350 ng/ml). This test is an indirect measurement of growth hormone. In general, IGF-1 will be low if free T is also low. This hormone decreases with age and its drop parallels the decrease in free T. Testosterone replacement stimulates IGF-1 and, therefore, growth hormone. Growth hormone has been called the hormone of youth because it causes the body to look younger and to increase muscle strength, muscle mass, hair growth, bone growth, and fat loss, and it's also an indirect measurement of leanness.

❑ Low IGF-1 (<150 ng/ml)

Treatment: We treat low IGF-1 with testosterone pellets, exercise, a high protein/low-carb diet, weight lifting, and weight loss. If the last four activities are undertaken without sufficient testosterone, IGF-1 will rarely increase in men over age fifty.

- The only reason IGF-1 might decrease during testosterone pellet treatment is if a patient loses weight. It goes back up when the patient's lean muscle mass to body fat ratio increases as the weight stabilizes.

- Head injuries can prevent IGF-1 from rising even when testosterone treatment is adequate, and then it must be replaced or stimulated with a hypothamlic growth hormone stimulator called peptides.

❏ High IGF-1 (>400 ng/ml)

- High IGF-1 may be transient and must be repeated under fasting conditions in the early morning to confirm a high level.

- If it's still elevated, an endocrinology consult is needed to rule out an adrenal or pituitary tumor secreting growth hormone.

❏ Elevated Prolactin (>23 ng/ml and less than 100ng/ml)

This is usually caused by exercise, oral estrogen replacement in women, methyl-dopa drugs, psychiatric medications, breast stimulation, use of marijuana, cocaine, opiates, or stress. If due to stress, the 8 a.m. cortisol will also be elevated. Moderately elevated prolactin can be treated by changing medications or making behavioral changes before retesting. Very high prolactin can be from a pituitary tumor (not cancer) and must be evaluated. Surgery is rarely required to treat this condition.

High prolactin can cause the testes to not function, causing testosterone production to fall. It also interferes with all sex hormones, preventing them from binding to receptor sites. When prolactin is elevated, all sex hormones decrease, and it appears as if the testicles are failing. Treatment with medication—dopamine agonists—can lower prolactin if the elevated levels aren't caused by a benign tumor. Sometimes when high prolactin is treated, no testosterone is needed, and the body becomes normal again.

Prolactin Level (3-200 ng/ml)

❏ Very Elevated Prolactin (200 ng/ml)

This very high level is usually caused by a benign microadenoma of the pituitary. This must be worked up and sometimes requires surgery or medication.

- [ ] Low Prolactin (<3 ng/ml)

This may indicate pituitary damage, dopamine drugs, or genetic low prolactin that causes poor attachment to loved ones. A neurosurgeon should be consulted.

LH and FSH

LH (leutenizing hormone) and FSH (follicle stimulating hormone) These pituitary hormones—LH and FSH—control the production of testosterone by the testes. LH stimulates the production of testosterone and sperm production. FSH is the primary hormone that stimulates sperm production.

- [ ] LH 1.5-6.0 MIU/L means normally working testes and *usually* means normal testosterone.
- [ ] LH <1.7 MIU/L without T replacement means pituitary or hypothalamic damage and the need for T or testicular stimulation.
- [ ] LH < 0.2 MIU/L means the man is on testosterone replacement or has had a pituitary abnormality. With a LH at this low level, when a man is on testosterone, he doesn't require treatment. If not, he needs testosterone.
- [ ] FSH 1.6-8.0 MIU/L means normally working testes with normal testosterone and normal sperm production.
- [ ] FSH < 1.5 MIU/L means a man is on testosterone replacement or has a pituitary abnormality.
- [ ] High LH, FSH: one or both LH > 9.3 MIU/L and FSH > 8.0 MIU/L

High LH and FSH occur when the testicles don't respond by making testosterone. The LH and FSH keep going up to get a normal T level, and if the testes fail from age, surgery, or

trauma, then these two hormones cause anxiety attacks and sleep disturbance since they peak at night.
Treatment is testosterone replacement with pellets.

Low LH and FSH can occur from damage to the pituitary that results in poor stimulation of the testes or from testosterone supplementation.
Treatment is either T replacement or HCG injections to stimulate the testes with a hormone (HCG) that looks and acts like LH.

Testing of Hormones from Non-Sex Glands in the Body: Cortisol, Thyroid, T3, T4, Reverse T3

Cortisol Testing (4-22.5 mcg/DL)

Cortisol is one of the adrenal hormones and is the key hormone we test to determine the normalcy of the adrenal gland. The normal range for cortisol is the same for both men and women of all ages. Testing must be in the morning, preferably after fasting and between 8 a.m. and 9 a.m. After that, the levels drop throughout the day, and it's hard to evaluate the normalcy of the blood levels. Cortisol is lowest between midnight and 3 a.m., during sleep.

❏ High Cortisol (>22.5 mcg/DL)

This is a sign of stress and can cause testosterone and estradiol to inactivate; elevate blood sugar; and cause weight gain, belly fat, depression, poor immune function, and fatigue.

- We treat high cortisol with Endo-Dren, an oral animal adrenal preparation, to suppress the production of cortisol in response to stressful circumstances.

- Very high cortisol may be caused by a pituitary tumor that produces the stimulating hormone ACTH, by an adrenal tumor, or by adult-onset adrenal hyperplasia.

❑ Low Cortisol (<4mcg/DL)

This causes severe fatigue, dizziness, weight loss, allergies, and low blood pressure. Low cortisol is treated with multiple doses of Endo-Dren. It can also be treated with prednisone or hydrocortisone. Cortisol usually becomes low after long-term stress or long-term use of steroid medication.

Thyroid Testing

Thyroid hormones regulate every cell in the body and manage the way each cell burns calories and makes energy. The thyroid slows down as we age, and we stop burning as many calories as we did when we were young. If we don't replace thyroid hormones, we get a weak heart, gain weight, swell up, sleep all the time, and go into a type of hibernation. Patients who take testosterone don't seem to improve with T pellets if their thyroid hormones are inadequate.

> **If we don't replace thyroid hormones, we get a weak heart, gain weight, swell up, sleep all the time, and go into a type of hibernation.**

Thyroid testing must be done first thing in the morning on an empty stomach with all medication withheld, even withhold thyroid meds. Men who take testosterone will not feel well unless their thyroid is in the normal range. Therefore, we monitor both testosterone and thyroid when we replace T for men. TSH is normal if it is less than <1 MIU/mL when a patient is on oral thyroid medicine. It can also be low if he has hyperthyroidism when on no thyroid medication; TSH is normal when it is less than 4.5 MIU/mL if a patient is not on thyroid medication.

We replace thyroid hormones in men who have low thyroid production, autoimmune thyroid dysfunction, and symptoms of hypothyroidism.

❑ TSH (thyroid stimulating hormone) 0.4-4.4 MIU/mL optimal level

TSH is the stimulating hormone produced by the pituitary gland and stimulates the thyroid. When we look at TSH, it's like indirectly looking at the thyroid gland. If the TSH is high, it's pushing the thyroid gland to make more thyroid hormones because it senses that the blood level is too low. TSH is inversely proportional to the activity of the thyroid gland.

❏ High TSH (>4.4 MIU/mL)

A high TSH level means that the thyroid is underproducing thyroid hormone. The thyroid is low. Thyroid replacement medication should be started.

❏ Low TSH (<0.4 MIU/mL)

Low TSH occurs when the TSH is suppressed by too much thyroid production in the body or by an antibody. It can also be low from thyroid hormone replacement.

❏ Free T3 and T4

The two active thyroid hormones are free T3 and free T4. We test for the free T3 and T4—the hormones without the binding protein—to evaluate the active portion of the thyroid hormone.

❏ Low Free T3 (<3.0 pg/dl)

This means you need more thyroid hormone replacement, like Cytomel® (liothyronine).

❏ High Free T3 (>4.5 pg/dl)

This means you either have too much thyroid replacement or have a hyperthyroid condition.

❏ Reverse T3 (<22 ng/dl optimal level)

Reverse T3 is an abnormal "shape" of the hormone T3 that cannot attach to receptor sites. Active T3 = Free T3 minus reverse T3. The higher the reverse T3, the lower the effective free T3 number is. If the free T3 value is normal and most of it is reverse T3, then your free T3 and free T4 numbers don't describe how you feel. Remember, we are treating based on symptom presentation as well as blood test results. The treatment for high reverse T3 is to give pure T3 to supplement the reverse T3 that isn't working. We make reverse T3 under the influence of stress and the hormone cortisol. When the levels of free T3 and free T4 don't match the symptoms, then getting a reverse T3 test makes sense to see if there really is enough T3 working.

❑ Low T4 free (<0.9 ng/dl)

This means you need thyroid replacement, or if you are on thyroid medication, you need a higher dose.

❑ High free T4 (>1.8 ng/dl)

This means you either have too much thyroid replacement or have a hyperthyroid condition. Low thyroid can be treated with thyroid replacement medication. Iodoral, a supplement that can stimulate the activity of the thyroid gland, can also be used with thyroid replacement, and can temporarily increase Free T4.

Blood Tests That Reflect Your Cardiac Health

The following abnormal lipid tests check for diseases and heart disease risk factors that may cause heart disease. In many cases, heart disease improves with T pellets and thyroid medication, as well as supplements.

❑ Elevated Total Cholesterol (>200 mg/dl or <5.2 mmol/L)

Total cholesterol is rarely a reliable measurement because it represents a combination of HDL (good) cholesterol and LDL (bad) cholesterol. I rarely take this number seriously when managing my patients.

❑ Low HDL (<46 mg/dl or 1.04-1.55 mmol/L)

HDL is the good cholesterol. It's important to raise a low HDL cholesterol count by taking niacin (a B vitamin) or fish oil

2,000-4,000 mg/day, or increasing aerobic exercise. If these supplements don't work, then the HDL level is genetic, and there is a question as to the negative impact of low HDL on heart disease.

❑ High LDL (>130 mg/dl)

LDL is the one lipid that can be associated with heart disease, and a high LDL can be treated with the following options:

- Replace testosterone with pellets
- Lower carbohydrates in the diet (not fats!)
- Increase regular aerobic activity
- Normalize thyroid with replacement of Iodoral® or thyroid supplement
- CoQ10 supplementation
- Red rice yeast at bedtime
- Statins when the previous methods don't work and a man has had evidence of heart artherosclerosis

❑ High Triglycerides (>150 mg/dl)

This comes from the consumption of carbohydrates and/or can be a genetic elevation or associated with diabetes and obesity. We treat high triglycerides with the following:

- Low-carb diet
- Aerobic exercise
- Weight loss
- Meformin ER 500 three times daily with food
- Victoza subcutaneous injections

❑ Elevated C-CRP (>3 mg/L)

This is a measure of whole body inflammation. Elevated C-CRP means that there is inflammation throughout the body that has spread from a single site or even multiple sites. Inflammation brings white blood cells to an area of trauma or disease to clean it up, so the body can heal. We all have inflammation at some time.

When inflammation occurs for long periods of time or is extreme in nature, it causes damage to the blood vessels of aging men. You can think of inflammation as the glue that circulates and causes the fat that is carried in the blood to stick to your arteries. This leads to atherosclerosis of the blood vessels and culminates in narrowed arteries and finally heart disease.

If your C-CRP is elevated for long periods of time, then finding the source of your inflammation is the key. The most common cause is a brief bacterial or viral infection, or it could be something more serious like an autoimmune disease (lupus, MS, or rheumatoid arthritis), an inflamed joint, obesity, or a malignancy. We find that oral gum disease is the most common cause of inflammation causing C-CRP to rise, so it's important to see your dentist if your C-CRP is elevated. If you can control your inflammation, then you can prevent arteriosclerosis, heart disease, and stroke.

Testosterone pellets are successful in suppressing inflammation in most cases and, therefore, they also help prevent heart disease.

Testosterone pellets are successful in suppressing inflammation in most cases and, therefore, they also help prevent heart disease.

All elevated C-CRP requires the following treatment, after confirmation with a repeat test.

Treatment for Elevated CRP:

- Receive testosterone pellets, if over age forty
- Take 81mg of aspirin daily (coated adult)

- Lose weight if your BMI is over 25
- Visit your dentist
- Take BioBalance® Health Curcumin supplement

❏ Elevated Homocysteine (>10.5 mmol/L)

This substance is one cause of heart attack, stroke, and Alzheimer's disease. High homocysteine in the blood is one of the "secret" cardiac and dementia risks. Unfortunately, it's not discussed with patients because doctors are so enamored with treating high cholesterol and statin therapy. It's like most cardiologists are under a spell that speaks "cholesterol…cholesterol" to them while they sleep, so they forget about the other risks.

Everyone makes homocysteine, but elevated levels occur when you're born with a genetic disease that worsens with age. Testosterone does not fix this problem; however, taking methylated B vitamins improves the condition and resolves the risk within six months. This treatment is lifelong.

High homocysteine is more dangerous than high cholesterol and is treatable with the correct type of vitamins, not expensive statin drugs that have many side effects. High homocysteine is related to the MTHFR genetic defect that causes stroke, heart disease, and blood clots.

Blood Tests That Reflect Your General Health

Many general health factors can affect how you respond to testosterone and how testosterone affects your general health. If you're healthy, testosterone generally improves your health. If you have certain problems or certain genetics, testosterone can negatively impact your health unless we intervene. Here's how we review your blood work.

Abnormal Metabolic Panel: Blood Glucose, Kidney Tests, Liver Function

The metabolic panel is really a group of blood tests for liver health, kidney function, and a blood sugar test. This is particularly important for patients starting testosterone replacement because the sex hormones are cleared from the body by the liver and kidneys. I have to make sure that the hormones I supplement can be metabolized out of the body when a man is finished with them.

❑ Elevated Glucose (>99 mg/dl)

This test indicates impending diabetes or AODM—Adult-Onset Diabetes Mellitus. Elevated triglyceride test results confirm the diagnosis. Abnormal blood sugar metabolism responds to metformin medication, diet, and exercise.

Treatment of elevated blood sugar (AODM) > 100 mg/dl to 130 mg/dl is pre-diabetes, and >131 mg/dl is Adult Onset Diabetes:

- Low-carb diet
- Aerobic exercise
- Six feedings daily with <25 grams of carbs per feeding
- Metformin 500 ER 2-3 daily with meals
- Victoza 0.6-1.8 mg sq daily
- Other oral diabetes drugs for blood sugars over 130

❑ Abnormal Kidney Function: High Creatinine >1.4 mg/dl and >107 mcmol/L, low GFR

This can be a simple case of dehydration or indicate a life-threatening problem that requires a complete medical evaluation. I repeat the test after hydration before I consider it a problem.

❑ Abnormal Liver Enzyme: Elevated Alkaline Phosphate >115 U/L

Repeat this test before further evaluation. If this enzyme is still elevated, then there's a problem with accelerated bone loss or abnormal liver function. This must be evaluated by your primary care physician to discover the reason for this abnormality. The good news is that T pellets stop bone loss and can bring the alkaline phosphate level back to normal if the problem is bone loss.

❑ Elevated Liver Enzymes: AST >40 U/L, ALT > 46 U/L

Repeat an elevated test before further evaluation. When these two enzymes are truly elevated, there is some damage to the liver that's causing the release of these enzymes. We worry about infection in the liver such as hepatitis, non-infectious fatty liver, or alcoholic liver damage. It is important to ascertain the cause and treat it appropriately.

Abnormal Complete Blood Count

The blood count test evaluates the number and size of red blood cells and white blood cells that are circulating at the time the blood is drawn. The counts are dependent on the patient's hydration, which varies from day to day; so if you get abnormal results, the test must be repeated to confirm a problem.

❑ High RBC (Red Blood Count) > 6.1 M/uL, Hemaglobin >17 g/dl, HCT (Hematocrit)>50%

A high red blood count can be due to a genetic cause that increases your absorption of iron from food. Too much iron and too many red blood cells can cause the blood to sludge and be difficult to push through the arteries, which puts a strain on the heart.

However, this test result can be elevated by factors other than genetic absorption, such as dehydration, viral and bacterial illness, and too much iron-containing vitamins or food.

There are two conditions that are diagnosed by discovering a high HB/HCT. The first is a genetic condition called erythrocytosis. These patients make too many red blood cells to begin with, and the number of red cells increases with smoking, high altitude, stress, and testosterone.

Erythrocytosis is a genetic disease that runs in some people with ancestry from Great Britain, France, Northern Germany, and the Netherlands. If we find that it's a genetic issue, we have men give blood every two to four months to rid themselves of excessive blood and iron.

The second condition is called hemochromatosis, which is indicated by a high RBC *and* high ferritin (see below). To diagnose it, we run the genetic test for hemochromatosis, and if that's negative we treat it like we treat erythrocytosis. If not, we ask a specialist to rule out any damage to the liver or other areas in the body and remove blood until the iron level is not dangerous.

If a man has either of these conditions, T supplementation of any kind can be harmful if they are not diagnosed and treated. So we look for it and treat it if necessary. Most men we diagnose with either problem have never been evaluated for it and can still take testosterone as long as we continue to monitor ferritin and high red blood cell counts.

❑ Elevated Ferritin (>290 ng/ml)

This is usually related to the genetic disease hemochromatosis, but sometimes this number is elevated because of overconsumption of alcohol. We must conduct a genetic test to diagnose hemochromatosis. If the test is positive, the treatment is blood donation two to four times a year to remove excess iron in order to avoid heavy metal damage to vital organs.

The treatments for a high blood count or high ferritin are as follows:

- Limit red meat, stop iron supplementation, stop all vitamin C supplements

- Donate blood often
- If HCT exceeds 50 percent, therapeutic phlebotomy (removal of blood) is necessary

Cancer Screening Tests

Prostate Cancer Screening Test (PSA):

- ❏ PSA test <3.5 ng/ml for ages up to 60 is normal (mainstream medical normal)
- ❏ % free PSA >25% is normal

The normal range increases with age.

Normal PSA Levels Increase With Age

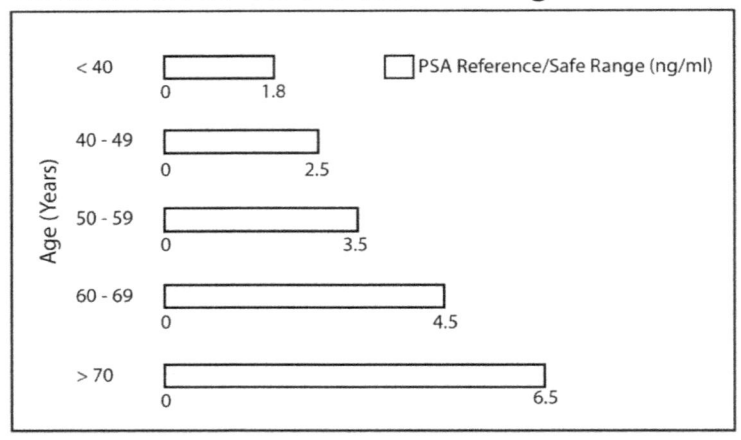

Age (Years)	PSA Reference/Safe Range (ng/ml)
< 40	1.8
40 - 49	2.5
50 - 59	3.5
60 - 69	4.5
> 70	6.5

Because a high level of PSA can be caused by other factors, we do a follow-up test. Men must comply with the following instructions thirty-six hours before the blood draw.

Pre-PSA Test Instructions:

- No sex
- No masturbation

- No exercise
- No hot tubs, steam rooms, etc.
- No rectal exams or anything in the rectum
- No use of allopurinol drug to treat gout

An elevated PSA test can indicate other conditions that are not cancer, such as benign prostatic hyperplasia (an enlarged prostate), trauma to the prostate, or prostate infection.

Some men who don't have prostate cancer have elevated PSAs for reasons we don't understand. There's no need to be upset about such a blood test value before it's evaluated by a urologist.

Remember this: Testosterone does not *cause* prostate cancer, but when prostate cells change to cancerous ones, they become sensitive to testosterone and grow faster. That's why we don't give testosterone to men who have untreated prostate cancer and those with advanced treated prostate cancer. However, if prostate cancer is removed or treated with radiation, many urologists are beginning to approve testosterone replacement after the cancer is treated. Some researchers believe testosterone prevents recurrence.

The Art and Science of Laboratory Interpretation

It's both an art *and* a science to interpret blood levels of hormones to determine whether a man is a candidate for testosterone replacement. It's not as simple as it seems. Because of the extensive training we receive, doctors have the ability to turn these test results into treatment plans that can save your health and life.

This chapter is meant *only* to give you an idea of what your lab results mean. It is not intended to replace the extensive knowledge of a physician. I

This chapter is meant *only* to give you an idea of what your lab results mean. It is not intended to replace the extensive knowledge of a physician.

spend a lot of time reeducating patients who get their lab results and make improper diagnoses for themselves. Self-diagnosis is not what this information is for. I offer it to you so that you realize that this is complicated stuff, and it's absolutely necessary to get this blood work to diagnose and treat testosterone deficiency.

CHAPTER 6

Sex and Testosterone: How It Works and What Can Go Wrong

This chapter has two distinct parts. The first is an examination of the *biological and physical issues* around sexual function. We examine the four parts of male sexual response, how it works, and what can go wrong. We also make recommendations that your health-care professional can use to help you find healthy medical interventions for your specific problems.

In the second part of this chapter, we look at what happens to *relationships* when libido, sexual function, or both are lost when T decreases, which can make sexual relations even more difficult. We explore how to repair the damage done to a man's sexual/loving relationship when the couple has struggled with the physical problems caused by testosterone deficiency. This is not to be taken lightly. Testosterone deficiency affects every area of a man's life, and it affects his partner, too.

BIOLOGICAL AND PHYSICAL ISSUES

The Truth About Sex and Testosterone

When I got married, I thought, "Great! We'll have sex every day! Just what I've always wanted!" I was only twenty-three back then, and I assumed that our sex life would be vibrant forever. But I was wrong. We had kids when my wife and I were in our thirties, which often meant we were too tired for sex.

But that wasn't the worst of it. In our forties, my wife told me she didn't want to have sex anymore. She said I could just forget it. I thought my life was over! I was still functioning well, and I couldn't believe this was the end of sex for me.

So I got a new car, worked late, exercised—anything to get rid of the sexual desire that hounded me. I guess that's what they call male menopause. It was terrible for our marriage.

But then I couldn't get it up anymore and I knew things couldn't get worse. What had happened to me? I was only fifty!"

Every day, this type of conversation takes place in doctors' offices all over the country. The typical medical response is, "Get used to it, buddy, because this is how it's going to be for the rest of your life" or "This is just normal for your age" or "Take Viagra®. It should help!"

At one time I worked exclusively with women, so I didn't fully realize that men go through as much pain and angst about losing their sexual ability as women do. Nor did I know that their feelings about it—just like women's—were routinely dismissed by medical professionals.

The truth is that the loss of libido hits men even harder than it does women. Most women seem able to accept the loss, but men are devastated if they can't function sexually.

The truth is that the loss of libido hits men even harder than it does women. Most women seem able to accept the loss, but men are devastated if they can't function sexually.

My message to men is this: you can absolutely get your vitality, sex drive, and sexual prowess back. You simply need an individualized treatment and a doctor who understands *all hormones*, not just testosterone. We can get you back in the game!

Testosterone Is the Answer

Here are some facts about T and sex:

- Testosterone is the foundation for a normal and spontaneous sex life. Without it, sex becomes mechanical.

- Sexual desire (libido) and erectile function are two separate aspects of male sexuality. Both are adversely affected by testosterone deficiency.

- You can get erections and even ejaculate with minimal testosterone if you use drugs like Viagra®. But only testosterone will affect your sex drive.

- There are four parts of sexual function: sex drive (libido), erectile function, ejaculatory function, and orgasm. Any of these can occur without the other, i.e., a man can have an orgasm without ejaculation or he can have an erection without having a sex drive. But satisfying sex that bonds a couple together requires as many of these four elements as is physically possible.

The Four Components of Sexual Function

Again, these are the four parts of sexual function:

- Sex drive, or libido
- Erectile function
- Ejaculation
- Orgasm

Sex Drive, or Libido

You know what this is. Your libido is what makes you want to have sex instead of watching a game on TV—or anything else! And your libido is literally all in your head because your sex drive comes from the parts of the brain that motivate sexuality, flirting, sexual fantasies, sexual dreams, foreplay, and the drive to have sex.

I can hear you thinking, *I thought my sex drive started with watching my partner undress, or when she or he touches me a certain way."* And you're right! You have peripheral nerves that send messages to your brain that get the gears turning. The brain, in fact, is actually your largest sex organ. But if it doesn't get enough testosterone or neurologic hormones, it can't produce the oxytocin needed to rev you up. Your brain hormones and neurotransmitters depend on testosterone to get things going.

I know I don't have to tell you that sex is important to all of us for many reasons. It produces the neurotransmitters that make us happy and motivates us to bond to others, so we can produce offspring and continue the species.

Humans are resilient, and we were created to survive in extreme environments. Think back to the caveman days. The sex drive stimulated them to create as many babies as possible so that the human race could withstand famine, drought, and other environmental disasters. Life spans were shorter back then. Just like other mammals, we stopped procreating and died when we were no longer fertile.

But now we live twice as long as is necessary to father children; and yet, our bodies still live by the old rules, and testosterone levels decrease at the same age as they did in caveman days. We live twice as long, but we can't sustain our testosterone production. So our sex drive disappears before we're ready to let it go.

My goal is to help you maintain both good health and optimum testosterone to enjoy life and sex as long as you draw breath. But there's one important issue that can prevent that, so let's address that now.

Erectile Function

You've heard a lot about erectile *dysfunction,* but not many people talk about erectile *function*. Erectile function has been described to me as a man's best friend; it's the morning wakeup call that pops up and makes you feel alive. It's that daily "something" that reassures you that you're still youthful and sexually capable. But when erections fail, a man loses confidence. He begins to feel *and act* old.

Guess what? It doesn't have to be that way. Testosterone is what creates the connection between a man's brain and his genitals, and I've witnessed the remarkable change that can take place in a man when his *erectile function* is restored. He becomes confident and self-assured again. Because I've seen how men transform so quickly, I now expect an emotional and personality miracle to occur after he gets testosterone pellets. There's much more benefit to regaining erectile function than simply fixing a sexual problem. It changes your quality of life.

> **There's much more benefit to regaining erectile function than simply fixing a sexual problem. It changes your quality of life.**

The Mechanics of Erections

A number of physiological functions must happen in the proper order for a man to get an erection and to maintain it long enough to orgasm, ejaculate, and please his partner. The two most necessary functions are that the pelvic arteries must dilate, and nitric oxide must be present to maintain the erection. In their book *The Science of Orgasm,* authors Barry Komisaruk, Carlos Beyer-Flores, and Beverly Whipple state that the whole process is so complicated that it's hard to believe that it happens automatically billions of time every minute across the world without anyone thinking about physiology or medicine. That is the beauty of sex: you don't have to think about it!

However, when erectile problems occur, doctors should consider all the necessary elements of erections: testosterone levels must be optimum; there must be adequate blood volume and heart activity; the autonomic nervous system must work to dilate the arteries and bring blood to the penis; and the circumstances must be such that a man can relax.

The first step in treating a man with ED is to replace his testosterone, but that's just the beginning. There are other factors that can cause ED, even when total testosterone and free testosterone are optimum.

Common Causes of Erectile Dysfunction:

- Aging
- Low testosterone
- Blood flow problems caused by diabetes and vascular disease (arteriosclerosis)
- High blood pressure, low blood pressure
- Smoking, drinking, and drug use
- Prescription medications
- Foods, such as coffee, that contain active vasoconstrictors
- Dehydration
- Obesity
- Genetic abnormalities that result in low T

The most common cause of ED is *aging*. As men age, their testosterone levels naturally drop. Most men wait a few years after their T levels drop to see a doctor—usually around age fifty-five. But in the past fifteen years, that pattern has changed, and we're now treating men in their forties who have ED.

Why? It's partly due to the chemicals in our environment that act as *estrogens* in men, blocking the T receptors throughout their bodies. Another major cause is the overwhelming percentage of American men who are obese. Obesity produces high levels of estrogen, which in turn, inactivate testosterone. Growth hormone and the estrogens found in milk and other foods also suppress testosterone production. The sad truth is that the modern male is slowly becoming infertile and impotent.

Environmental Causes of ED:

- By-products of industry that contaminate what we eat and the air we breathe
- Heavy metals in the environment: Mercury in fish, lead and aluminum to mention a few.

The Aging Process

In the aging process, the first falling domino is the loss of *testosterone*, which triggers a decrease in *growth hormone*, after which *cholesterol* (total and LDL) increases. To counter that, a man is usually prescribed statins to reduce his cholesterol, which reduce testosterone even further!

The result is that the man loses muscle and gains belly fat, which binds up his testosterone and inactivates it. An obese man becomes insulin resistant (prediabetic), and so he gains even more weight. Because he lacks muscle mass and stamina, he becomes even more inactive, eats junk food to self-medicate, becomes depressed, drinks more alcohol, gains more weight, and his ED becomes worse. His primary care physician offers him Viagra® so he can have sex, but nothing is done to correct his initial problem of lost testosterone!

The ED Approach

> **Most of our patients require testosterone replacement to achieve a healthy sex drive and to become sexually active again.**

Most of our patients require testosterone replacement to achieve a healthy sex drive and to become sexually active again. So, we treat them first with testosterone (which restores the libido), then adjust the medications they take to control other medical issue like high blood pressure or diabetes, and then we put them on a plan to lose weight. Daily exercise is crucial to improve blood flow throughout the body.

Finally, if ED is still an issue, I add Viagra® or Cialis®, which may be necessary if the patient has had low T for a long time, as some irreversible changes may have occurred that inhibit blood flow. However, Viagra® may not work if the patient takes blood pressure medication or if his blood vessels have stiffened or severely narrowed. The old drug metformin ER is now used to dilate old, stiff vessels.

> ### Erectile Dysfunction: Harbinger of Future Heart Disease
>
> Erectile dysfunction is an early warning sign of impending cardiovascular problems. ED usually shows up about five years before a man experiences a stroke or heart attack and should be considered a sign of impending heart and vascular disease. So far, traditional medicine treats only the symptom—vascular narrowing—with Viagra®, and there's no follow-up to investigate the source of the problem. But if we *regard ED as an early warning sign for future disease*, we can document vascular atherosclerosis, change the man's diet, and increase his exercise, as well as use supplements like Neo40®, a vascular roto-rooter and vascular dilator, to improve the flexibility and patency of his arteries.

Medical Problems, Medications, and ED

If your total T and free T are normal—or your testosterone has been fully replaced and you still have ED—then you'll need your doctor's help to look into other medical problems that may be the root of the problem.

There are a variety of medical causes that can lead to ED, and they can be ruled out by getting extensive blood tests, blood flow studies of the pelvis, an ultrasound of the heart and vascular system, a doppler, or a calcium CT scan. Through a process of elimination, these tests can either confirm or rule out your cause or causes of ED.

There are a lot of things that can compromise your testosterone levels. Simply entering the hospital for an operation can lower your total and free T blood levels, although temporarily. Chronic diseases including diabetes, vascular disease (atherosclerosis), low blood pressure, heart failure, pituitary disease, and a history of mumps. And any medical problem that causes fatigue can decrease both free T and libido.

Sadly, even the medications and treatments for disease can reduce a man's testosterone. These include radiation of the pelvis, chemotherapy, pelvic or prostate surgery, and certain blood pressure medications. For example, men who have high blood pressure and are taking antihypertensive medications in the form of beta blockers, diuretics, and ACE inhibitors can experience erectile dysfunction caused by their medications.

Face it, if you don't feel well, you're not going to feel frisky or want sex like you would if you were healthy. That's why, in my practice, we look at the whole picture. We treat as many contributing medical diseases as we're qualified to treat, so we can change our patients' medications to those that don't damage either their libido or their erectile function.

Lifestyle and ED

Many things in a man's daily life—including his habits, activities, and the substances he ingests—can cause ED. But there are no warning labels to tell you that these things are hazardous to your erections! So I've compiled a list of things that can cause a man to lose his ability to have sex, which you'll find on page 143 of this chapter.

Jerry, a forty-seven-year-old plumber, came to me because of ED and a lack of sex drive. He had low free T and several other minor medical issues that could affect his ability to get and keep a rigid erection. He was obviously fit, with well-defined muscles, despite his low free T, which is not typical of my patients' pre-pellet body type. I decided to treat him with pellets after unsuccessfully attempting to increase his free T and lower his estrogens with Arimidex®.

Jerry was very motivated to get better because he and his wife had always enjoyed a very active sex life, sometimes having sex more than once a day. The loss of this form of connection was damaging his marriage.

Finally, after several office visits where I exhausted all of my options to resolve his ED, his wife mentioned a weird habit he had that she thought might "mean something." Jerry drank Monster Energy caffeine drinks all day long and then took a highly caffeinated power drink before he worked out every night. When he got home, he couldn't perform. Eureka! That was the problem—caffeine!

Remember that an erection requires the blood vessels to dilate in order to become rigid. Caffeine does the opposite; it constricts blood vessels.

Caffeine is a vasoconstrictor and, when taken in large amounts, it causes impotence. (One Monster Energy drink has 160 mg of caffeine, and his energy power drink had 360 mg of caffeine.) Remember that an erection requires the blood vessels to dilate in order to become rigid. Caffeine does the opposite; it constricts blood vessels.

Some men are more sensitive to caffeine than others, but one of the first things a man should do when faced with ED is to wean off caffeine! Over the next two months, Jerry backed off from all caffeine except two cups of coffee a day. Voila! His erections were back! If you take this approach, remember that caffeine withdrawal is a painful process, so be sure to wean off it slowly.

Through this process, Jerry also discovered that his low sex drive wasn't due to a lack of T. It came from his fear that he wouldn't be able to perform. That, too, resolved itself. In the end, he didn't need T pellets!

There are other vasoconstrictors found in foods and drugs, and if you have uncontrolled high blood pressure, some of these substances can be deadly. In the list below of foods and drugs to avoid, vasoconstrictors are noted by an asterisk (*).

Foods and Drugs to Avoid That Can Cause ED:

- ADD and ADHD medicines / amphetamines*
- Adrenal supplements
- Angiotensin*
- Anti-androgen drugs (Proscar®, finasteride, Propecia®)
- Antipsychotics
- Asthma medications and inhalers
- Caffeine in excessive amounts
- Cocaine*
- Cold medications / antihistamines*/ Sudafed®*
- Diet pills (both prescribed and over the counter)*
- Dopamine (L-Dopa)
- Epinephrine* / adrenaline*
- Green tea
- Nicotine
- Methylphenidate*
- Phenylephrine*
- Prednisone, cortisone
- Sudafed, pseudoephedrine*

Remember what your high school science teacher taught you: For every action, there is an equal and opposite reaction. And in the world of substances and drugs, that's true. If you take the medications above, you may very well lose your erections.

If you want to improve your erection, you can incorporate the following substances and medications that relax the blood vessels.

Vasodilators That Can Help Treat ED:
- Nitric oxide (Neo40®-supplement)
- Viagra®, Levitra®, Cialis®
- Magnesium supplements
- L-arginine and ornithine
- Diazoxide*
- Minoxidil®*
- Antiseizure medication
- Nitroglycerine

Always consult your physician before using any of these medications for ED. Exercise, deep breathing, and yoga are natural remedies that can help treat ED too.

Blood Pressure Medicine

Yes, high blood pressure and low blood pressure can cause ED, so the blood pressure medicine you take is very important. It must deliver a normal blood pressure, not low blood pressure, not less than 110/70.

The best blood pressure medications to take are ARBs (angiotensin receptor blockers) such as Benicar® (olmesartan) and calcium-channel blockers like Cardizem® (diltiazem Hcl).

The worst blood pressure drugs for your ED are lisinopril (angiotension converting enzyme inhibitor, or ACE inhibitor) and Lopressor®, Toprol XL® (metoprolol) and Procardia® (nifedipine), all beta blockers. Diuretics like HCTZ (hydrochlorothiazide),

Lasix® (furosemide), and Maxzide® (triamterene-HCTZ) also lower blood volume and can decrease erection firmness and erection longevity. If the only blood pressure medication that works for you is one of these, then continue to take it. You can add testosterone, Viagra®, or other meds to help with your ED.

Anti-Inflammatory Meds: Motrin, Advil, Hydrocortisone, and Anti-Prostaglandins

Most people take over-the-counter or prescription medications to treat aches and pains and reduce inflammation. However, high doses, daily dosing, and prescription anti-inflammatory medications can decrease the prostaglandins that are needed to create an erection.

Anti-inflammatory medicines are rarely the primary cause of ED, but they can contribute to it. If you anticipate that you'll have sex, just skip a dose.

Recreational Drugs and ED

Recreational drugs are illicit, as are illegal drugs obtained without a doctor's prescription. The categories are marijuana; cocaine/ecstacy/methamphetamines; heroin; and morphine. These drugs decrease your sex drive and the ability to get an erection.

Cocaine, ecstacy, and methamphetamines constrict the blood vessels to the pelvis. Conversely, they're also known to intensify orgasm—and they do—if you can ever get an erection. Over time, they cause loss of orgasm and ED. Opiates like heroin and morphine kill the sex drive.

Marijuana (THC) can cause a low sex drive as well as ED, because it elevates prolactin levels and, in turn, increases estrogen blood levels. A good rule of thumb is that if you're getting man boobs, then you have too much estrogen and should slow down or stop your use of THC.

The recent legalization of marijuana in several states has opened the door to the development of specialized strains of marijuana that have fewer adverse sexual effects and more of the good anti-anxiety results. We see fewer side effects from these strains, so there's hope that the new forms of legalized marijuana may be used in the future without exposing the patient to other medical problems and ED.

There's another component of the hemp plant that doesn't cause ED: CBD. CBD is from the male hemp plant and does not have active THC as a component. It's the medicinal portion of the hemp plant that doesn't cause increases in prolactin or estrogen, so there's no ED associated with its use. I sometimes recommend that my patients take CBD to relax, to help drop their blood pressure to normal without using other drugs, and for insomnia.

Anabolic Steroids = Adrenal Androgens

My advice: stay away from these completely. If you've previously self-medicated with adrenal steroids, illegal androgens, or mixtures of drugs from outside the US to enhance your physical performance, you may now have testicular failure (no T production) as well as adrenal failure (Addison's disease). If that's the case, you'll need to replace all your adrenal hormones and your testosterone. Addison's disease is a complicated disease that should be treated by an endocrinologist.

Men who habitually use adrenal steroids to enhance their sexual performance when they already make their own adequate testosterone are inviting danger.

Men who habitually use adrenal steroids to enhance their sexual performance when they already make their own adequate testosterone are inviting danger and will spend at least half their lives consumed with doctor visits.

Dehydration

If you want to get an erection, your blood volume must be close to normal, which means that you need to drink *water or noncaffeinated liquids* to fill up your blood volume "tank." If you drink alcohol, travel on an airplane, sweat, or exercise, you can become dehydrated. So pay attention to your life activities before you have sex!

Of course, exercise is good for you. It lowers blood pressure and dilates your blood vessels, but you must provide enough blood volume to avoid ED. That means you should drink eight eight-ounce glasses of water per day—and that's if you aren't doing anything physical. Double that if you exercise. When you exercise, you also need to preserve your electrolytes, salt, and potassium, so it's wise to drink Gatorade G2 when you exercise.

Stress

The stress of modern life can't be avoided; however, it doesn't have to control you. Long working hours, fear of financial insecurity, and the constant intrusion of text messages and phone calls increase your cortisol, estrone, and adrenalin. These are the hormones that bind up your testosterone and can prevent you from getting an erection.

It's important to have time to yourself when you can relax, turn off your phone, and enjoy life. Figure out what you enjoy that allows you to relax and have fun, and then schedule it as part of your day. Aerobic exercise, weight lifting, stretching, yoga, reading, sitting and watching TV, or playing golf are all ways to chill out your adrenal gland and get your sex life back on track.

Sedentary Lifestyle

Most of us use our brains more than our bodies, so we sit around making fat out of our food. And fat makes estrogen. In men, too much estrogen counteracts testosterone and results in impotence. The fatter a man is, the worse the problem!

If you have a sedentary lifestyle, you're not using your muscles enough and, therefore, your blood flow to all parts of the body is inhibited. Further, this causes a decrease in nitric oxide—a critical component necessary to getting an erection. You can't just sit every day and expect to have a great sex life. Get up and get moving!

Veganism

I'm not a fan of veganism—eliminating animal protein from a diet—not just because I'm a confirmed omnivore (I eat everything), but because my vegan patients don't have the education they need to know what they should eat every day to provide their bodies with the vital proteins required for optimum body function.

Vegan men often end up lacking muscle mass and necessary hormones because they don't know how to ingest the proper amount of plant protein needed to replace meat, cheese, eggs, and other animal products that provide amino acids for bodily functions.

Don't discount this shortfall. All stimulatory hormones, to every gland, are made of proteins, and ED can result from a lack of nitrous oxide, which comes from meat proteins.

> **I have rarely met a man who properly nourishes himself through veganism.**

I have rarely met a man who properly nourishes himself through veganism. But even then, his muscle mass is often low and weak because he lacks the building blocks of animal proteins. The worst form of veganism is when a man eats a salad every day and all the junk food he can ingest! To have adequate sex hormones and nitric oxide, you need to eat a balanced diet that includes eggs, cheese, and some meat.

Smoking

Tobacco contains nicotine, and nicotine is a vasoconstrictor. It results in hypoxia—lack of oxygen—throughout your body. One cigar is equal to a pack of cigarettes, so you can't deny that you're a smoker if you smoke cigars!

I've known several long-term smokers who continued to smoke and were then angry that they became completely impotent, so much so that Viagra® didn't work. So if the fear of losing your life hasn't motivated you to quit smoking, then quit to save your sex life!

Inherited Diseases

Genetic inherited factors that cause ED cannot be cured, but they can usually be treated. The man with a genetic profile that leaves him with very low testosterone can be successfully treated with testosterone pellets. Take Klinefelter syndrome—an XXY male chromosomal abnormality where a man has an extra X chromosome—for example. This inherited genetic disease usually presents early after puberty and results in low blood levels of free T, infertility, and ED.

These boys are usually diagnosed early in their lives because their bodies look obese and have belly fat. They are late to go through puberty, if they do at all.

We treat these adolescents and men who have the syndrome with testosterone pellets to achieve high normal T levels. And they enjoy excellent results! They're transformed from young men with no muscle mass and plentiful belly fat into normally functioning and very masculine-looking men. Although they can rarely produce sperm, it's possible for them to have a normal sex life.

One problem in treating these boys is that there's no medical specialty that concentrates on their problem. Pediatricians are afraid of testosterone replacement, and even if they do administer it, they usually don't give young men enough to become fully male. Even urologists don't know what to do with them. That's why I stepped in. I've successfully treated several young men with this condition who are grateful and very satisfied with their transformation.

Hormone Deficiencies and Imbalances

- Low thyroid
- Low or high cortisol

- Low GH
- Low FSH, Low LH
- Low ACTH (adrenocorticotropic hormone)

Hormone deficiencies or hormonal imbalances can be the cause of reversible ED and infertility. Deficiency of the hormones—thyroid, cortisol, growth hormone, and the pituitary hormones FSH, LH, and ACTH—can cause sexual dysfunction. Therefore, we check all the hormones that can be replaced at the same time we check for testosterone deficiency.

Hormone Overproduction

- Estradiol
- Estrone
- Prolactin
- Cortisol

Overproduction of other hormones like estradiol, estrone, prolactin, and cortisol can inactivate testosterone and single-handedly cause ED. These problems are diagnosed through blood work, and then we balance them either by using medications or by replacing these hormones to normal levels.

Trauma to the Brain or Testicles

Trauma to the brain or testicles can cause damage to the organs that are vital to sexual response. This type of trauma can immediately cause testosterone deficiency, or there can be a delayed response that presents itself as the victim ages.

Brain trauma of any kind—such as that sustained from football, boxing, or participating in other contact sports—can cause post-traumatic brain injury, which can affect both the brain's stimulation of the sex hormones as well as the libido. Auto accidents can also cause brain trauma and, in turn, have an impact on how much testosterone a man can produce.

Head trauma that involves the pituitary and hypothalamus can adversely affect the stimulation of testosterone and other sex hormones by the pituitary. This small gland is located behind the bridge of the nose, and trauma to that area of the brain can cause deficiencies in many other glands, including the testicles, thyroid, and adrenal gland.

Surgery or radiation around or involving the pituitary gland or hypothalamus can stunt production of all hormones, but the ones that affected men miss the most are growth hormone and testosterone. If brain surgery or radiation of the brain is administered before puberty, not only will a boy's normal sexual organs and hormones not mature, his growth will be stunted as well from the lack of growth hormone. It's imperative that these hormones be replaced in sufficient amounts so that these boys can become men.

Abe came to see me for the first time when he was twenty-nine. He was accompanied by his girlfriend and was cheerful, despite all the medical care he'd endured.

Abe had been diagnosed with a brain tumor prior to puberty. It involved his pituitary gland and the hypothalamus, and radiation was the only treatment available at the time. He was told that he would be given growth hormone and testosterone after radiation, so he'd achieve a normal stature and male development. But now, at twenty-nine, he stood only 5 feet 4 inches tall and had ED.

His cancer treatment was successful and he lived. But he was never given growth hormone, even though the part of his brain that produced growth hormone was gone. The amount of testosterone he was given was miniscule compared to what a normal adolescent needs to fully develop. Because he was treated at a teaching hospital, his doctors changed as frequently as their rotations, and there was no continuity to his care. Everyone had promised him growth hormone, but no one ever prescribed it. He told me how he continually asked for growth hormone until, one day, a new doctor told him it was too late. His growth plates had sealed, he was no longer able to grow.

Abe came to me to receive the testosterone he needed to be sexually active and "whole" again. Abe did well, and he and his girlfriend have found what they needed to treat his ED. However, his treatment will need to change if he wants to father children. I'll have to send him to a fertility doctor at that time. But Abe will be on testosterone pellets for the rest of his life.

Treatment of ED for the Average Guy

It's difficult to recommend a single treatment for all men who have ED, because, as you've read, everyone is different. But I'd like to offer a typical treatment plan that can bring the majority of men back to sexual wholeness!

In general, aging men who experience erectile dysfunction should consider the following treatment steps as they discuss their condition with their physician:

- Replace lost testosterone *using the pellet method only.* No other delivery form of testosterone replacement will be as effective.

- Change antihypertensive medicine to Cardizem® or Benicar®.

- Normalize your blood sugar as much as possible. If you're diabetic, you need to be on an ACE inhibitor or an angiotensin receptor blocker (ARB) for your kidneys to increase the glomerular filtration rate in your kidneys. Saving your kidneys trumps treating ED.

- Change any beta blockers and ACE inhibitors to other antihypertensives if possible.

- If you have atherosclerosis, you'll have a complicated treatment including anti-inflammatory medicine and Neo40® to dilate pelvic blood vessels. Then we'll finally

- treat the symptom of ED with Cialis® 2.5 mg/day, daily low-dose aspirin, along with weight loss and/or statins, and you'll possibly get stints in the iliac arteries to increase blood flow. Daily Cialis® currently costs about four hundred dollars per month.

- Other strategies for treating ED symptoms include phosphodiesterase inhibitor type 5, Cialis®, Levitra®, and Viagra® (generic Viagra® currently selling for eight dollars per pill (100 mg)).

- In addition, you should consider taking the supplement L-arginine/ornithine in order to increase the nitrous oxide in your blood stream and Neo40®, which increases the nitric oxide and dilates your blood vessels enough to lower blood pressure. It also increases the blood flow to the penis. Both supplements are available without prescriptions, and compared to Viagra®-like drugs, they are reasonably priced.

Ejaculation Issues

ED is not the only problem that can occur when men age and their testosterone levels drop. Abnormal ejaculation—and even no ejaculation at all—is the second-most complained-about issue. And don't confuse lack of ejaculate with a lack of orgasm. Orgasm doesn't always result in ejaculation. They are two completely different physiologically complicated sexual responses.

Ejaculations normally measure 2cc to 5cc, although some men ejaculate more in their prime. The ejaculate is composed of sperm and liquid from the testicles, prostate fluid, and fluid from the vasdeferens and epididimus. Each organ contributes one-third of the ejaculate. When a man gets a vasectomy, the third that comes from the testicles is blocked off, so the volume of ejaculate decreases by about 30 percent.

Dry Ejaculation (little or no ejaculation)

Testosterone stimulates the other two sources of fluid. However, when men age, a loss of fluid occurs because the amount of nitric oxide secreted from all the sexual tissues that contribute to ejaculate decreases. Other causes of low-volume ejaculation include dehydration and medications that cause vasoconstriction. Adding testosterone can increase the volume somewhat, but sometimes it must be augmented by Arginine/ornithine supplement and Neo40® to get any appreciable volume increase.

Delayed Ejaculation

Testosterone makes successful sex possible, but it has little to do with the timing of ejaculation. Some guys can train themselves to have sex for hours (if they can keep an erection that long), and they orgasm and ejaculate when they choose to. But that's not what men complain about. The problem is when they have sex for a prolonged period of time and can't ejaculate or finish the act. It leaves them "hanging," so to speak.

Delayed ejaculation is most often caused by antidepressants, but it's sometimes the result of a man having trained himself to delay ejaculation, either for birth control reasons or for the pleasure of his partner. If repeated on a regular basis, delaying ejaculation can become a habit that's difficult to break. When this happens, I recommend counseling and behavioral modification.

Premature Ejaculation

Men are often reluctant to discuss their sexual performance or their sexual dysfunction with anyone, especially a doctor. It's not easy to talk about sex with anyone, including a sexual partner. For some reason, most men feel the most secretive about premature ejaculation but, of course, it's something their partner is well aware of.

Men get a lot of their information from their buddies, and because they're competitive, they compare themselves with their friends. They would never mention their premature ejaculation problem to other men, but they hear the stories other men tell about *their* sexual prowess and then compare themselves to those stories. So, they may feel like they don't quite measure up in the sexuality department, whether they do or not!

Men can be plagued by the myth of the iconic western hero of movies, novels, and TV shows. You know what that is—the tough, strong, silent type that's become the model for masculinity. And they have expectations of themselves as providers and defenders and tough guys. It's important to bring home the bacon, make sure their families are safe, and provide for them in all the ways they can. But they can never cry or show weakness—or at least they may think so.

So, if you're striving to be all the things that make up a "real" man, what happens when you can't maintain an erection more than a few minutes without ejaculating? It reminds you of when you were an inexperienced teenager and got so excited you couldn't hang on for more than a few minutes. You feel weak and immature, not exactly like what the cowboys portrayed.

Taking antidepressants is the accepted medical treatment for premature ejaculation, but it's the very same drug treatment that causes other problems for men without premature ejaculation. Counseling can also help the relationship while you deal with the issue. You can't continually leave your partner in a state of arousal and frustration. So do explore other options to sexually satisfy your partner in ways other than intercourse. Testosterone pellets also help, but not completely. Even though this image is totally unrealistic, men still seem to believe it!

Orgasm

An orgasm is the peak of sexual excitement and is sometimes, but not always, accompanied by ejaculation. Orgasm is the release from sexual tension. At climax, the libido is diminished, which decreases the arousal that led to sexual behavior.

Even though there are muscle contractions and physical signs of orgasm in the body, orgasm is primarily experienced in the brain. In contrast, ejaculation is focused in the urethra (the tube from your bladder through your penis). The feeling of urethral release is also pleasant, but it doesn't have to be part of orgasm for you to feel the release from sexual tension.

What happens to the body during orgasm? You might be surprised, but it's all in your head! In general, the whole brain lights up on an MRI. The heart rate and respiratory rate increase, and there's an increase in blood flow to the pelvis. The hormone oxytocin, from the posterior pituitary, stimulates penile secretions, and dopamine increases erections. The feeling of bonding increases, and prolactin surges at the point of climax, which decreases libido and increases sexual satisfaction and bonding. The study of orgasm is an ever-developing specialty in medicine, and the actual map of an orgasm has not yet been plotted at the time of this writing.

At orgasm, your entire body usually experiences some spasmodic muscular contraction, and your state of desire dissipates—at least for a while. For most, an orgasm is accompanied by a visible release of the fluid called ejaculate. But, as previously mentioned, these are separate aspects of the sexual conclusion experience, and one or more may be absent at orgasm.

The following drugs block orgasm:

- Antipsychotics (anything that blocks dopamine)
- Antidepressants that increase serotonin (SSRIs)
- Antidepressants tricyclic
- Amphetamines and cocaine

If you must take antidepressants or antianxiety medications, choose Wellbutrin®, mirtazapine, or trazodone.

Remember: A man can have an orgasm without an erection or ejaculation. He can also ejaculate without an erection. Finally, a man can have an erection without an ejaculation or an orgasm but be satisfied because he satisfied his partner.

Changes in the Sexual Experience as Men Age

In *The Science of Orgasm,* the authors describe the four changes in erection, ejaculation, and orgasm that occur with aging. These are consistent with what I hear from my patients before they're treated with testosterone.

The four changes are:

- The penis requires more direct stimulation to become erect.
- The tone of the erection is not as firm as when the man was young.
- The force of ejaculation is less, and the volume is diminished.
- It takes longer to ejaculate, and the refractory period—the time between erections—lengthens.

If testosterone is replaced early on when the testosterone drops (usually between the ages of forty and fifty-five), replacing testosterone with or without a drug like Viagra® will normally reverse the first two issues. Diminished ejaculate and the length of the refractory period, however, are rarely reversible with testosterone.

But on the positive side, as men age, they tend to slow down their love-making, and they pay more attention to their partner than they did when they were young and in a hurry. Learning new ways to make your partner happy and then trying them out can lead to more satisfying sex than when the goal was simply to rush to orgasm.

RELATIONSHIP ISSUES

Our patients come to my co-author Brett Newcomb and me when they're in a crisis and they need hormones or they need counseling. The material in this second part of the chapter describes Brett's approach to working with couples in crisis.

Brett's Story

When I was thirty-eight years old, I met and married my wife, who was ten years younger than me. For the next decade, we lived an idyllic life. We travelled, we camped, we worked hard, and we played hard. Our relationship was intensely satisfying on every level.

When Phyllis was thirty-eight, we decided to start a family. We didn't want to get older only to pursue "more"; we wanted to dedicate our lives to having and raising children. But getting pregnant was easier said than done. We tried and eventually underwent fertility treatments. Nothing worked.

But then a strange and, to us, miraculous thing happened. We were contacted by an attorney who didn't actually know us—he knew of us. He asked if we'd consider adopting a baby. We went through that grueling process and at the end, we had a beautiful, healthy baby boy.

Just as Phyllis turned forty, tragedy struck when her father was diagnosed with ALS (Lou Gehrig's disease). He remained at home, and we helped take care of him there until he died a little over a year later. During his illness, Phyllis spent as much time taking care of him as she could. At the same time, she was a full-time teacher and had a three-year-old son. I was also teaching and building my career as a private-practice counselor. Phyllis carried most of the load, making our family work and caring for her dad until his death.

A couple of years later, it was obvious that Phyllis's grandmother could no longer live alone; so we built an addition on our house and she moved in with us. She wanted to die at home, not in some institution or care facility, and she lived with us for three years.

Phyllis retired from teaching and became her primary caregiver until she died.

During this ten- to twelve-year period, Phyllis's body had changed. As she aged, she'd lost her testosterone and, along with that, her libido. She had zero sex drive. Concerned, she talked to her gynecologist, and he told her that this was common for women her age who'd experienced the type of intense stress that Phyllis had undergone. "As you get old, you lose interest in sex." That was his message. He said there was nothing medically wrong with her body; she was just at "that time of life," and we needed to learn to deal with it.

While Phyllis was going through the normal process that women experience when they go through menopause, the stress from her responsibilities to take care of elderly relatives and to raise a child was extreme. At the end of this cycle, Phyllis had changed. Life had changed her and had changed for her. She was still an angel, but she was different.

Yet I was the same. I had my same, normal sex drive—and I felt like I was starving. As I began to grapple with these changes in our life, I started to concentrate on the sexual cuing that went on between us. Was I clearly signaling that I wanted to have sex? Was I using cues that had worked for us before, to which she had regularly responded? Did I need to learn to adapt my style to this new reality? What other ways could I signal her of my interest?

One tool I frequently use in communication is humor. So I started to make jokes about putting a "Yes!" or "No!" sign on our headboard, so I'd know whether sex was in the cards that night. I teased that if I just knew what lay ahead, I'd be less likely to get my feelings hurt or to get angry. We both understood the joke, but it actually wasn't funny. And it didn't work.

As it turned out, I was the only one who ever turned the card over to signal an interest in sex. Phyllis was never interested because her libido was gone. I didn't know that at the time, so I pushed harder. Then I felt rejected and got my feelings hurt over and over again. I played mental games with myself being victimized by her loss of interest. I accused her of never initiating sex, which was true. Her *answer was that she never thought about it; but she said that if I let her know when I was in need, she'd comply.*

I started keeping track of how frequently we had sex and how often I'd tried and failed to get her attention. It became impossible to communicate about this topic honestly—at least for me. I played manipulative games and set up elaborate strategies to try to trick her into feeling sexual desire. Of course, that never worked because the issue was hormonal, not relational.

I found myself trying to be "in control" and told myself that I wouldn't approach her for sex until she came to me with intimacy in mind. That didn't work either. My body would fight my attempt at control, and I'd find myself asking for sex yet again. Phyllis always responded lovingly, but my ego couldn't stand it. I got angry and acted out.

One of my coping strategies was to dive headlong into my work. I thought if I was busy at the office and hardly ever home, there'd be less opportunity to notice the change that had taken place there. So I worked more and more, made more money, and took on more commitments—in large measure because it hurt so much to be home and not be desired.

Part of how we survived for that year or so was a strategic rhythm that we'd developed. I'd be in denial and struggle to not need intimacy because I didn't want to have to ask for Phyllis's attention. But then I'd get moody and angry. I became an incredibly good pouter. When I pouted and acted angry, she'd eventually realize that the solution was to initiate sex with me, and for a while I'd be "all better."

After those episodes, I always felt ashamed and angry with myself. Why couldn't I be more in control of myself? Why couldn't I understand that this was natural and that we loved each other, but that sex was no longer in the picture? Was there something I could do to minimize my own desire?

There seemed to be no solution. I began to think that I had only two options: I could either have an affair (a friend with benefits) or get a divorce. But I didn't want to divorce Phyllis. I wanted to spend my life with her, but I simply couldn't live without sex. And I couldn't be dishonest or betray her trust in me. Trust is such a fragile and easily broken thing, and having Phyllis's trust had always been one of the most important parts of our relationship to me. I was afraid. I didn't want to be this person; I didn't want to create a crisis because I couldn't control my libido. I was desperate.

Then I found Dr. Maupin. She and I began to work together professionally, sharing clients who were having emotional and physical problems that were damaging their lives and destroying their relationships. She treated the physical problems, and I treated the emotional. As I worked with Dr. Maupin and learned about how testosterone replacement rejuvenated women, I began to think this might be the solution to our problem. I asked Phyllis to make an appointment to see if her aging issues and loss of libido could be reversed. Was it possible that Phyllis's regular doctor had been wrong and something physical was at the core of our problems?

The answer was "yes"! But by the time we got Phyllis's body adjusted, I started to have my own libido issues due to aging and the resulting testosterone loss. The aging cascade had been triggered for me as well. God really must have a sense of humor!

We've both been blessed to have found Dr. Kathy Maupin, who taught us about testosterone loss and how damaging it can be to relationships and to our health. She replaced our hormones that were out of balance as a result of aging and the very high stress levels we'd experienced. We are now, thankfully, back in balance and back in rhythm with each other. I can't thank her enough for saving our health and our relationship.

When couples are in sync sexually and their rhythms match, that's an ideal situation. But if those rhythms begin to drift apart, you sometimes need to take a step back to recognize that something has changed. Both partners will eventually notice that sex has become ritualized (sex only on Saturday morning, for example). For a while you may think it's due to a busy schedule, demands of the children and their schedules, work responsibilities that exhaust you, chores around the house that need to be done, and more. But eventually you notice that sex is not exciting, mutually desired, or readily enjoyable any more.

The biggest disaster in a man's life is when he can no longer have sex with the person he loves. This issue causes more divorces, affairs, and emotional pain than any other. By the time the couple reaches out for help, the blame game has already been established and the negative games have begun. This is when Dr. Maupin and I step in to find a way to heal not just one person, but both individuals and the relationship itself.

The first issue is to stop the finger-pointing, so the healing can begin. It's possible that neither party is to blame, and that aging and the associated changes are the real culprits. It's entirely possible, indeed likely, that neither partner has lost interest in or stopped *loving* the other; it may be that one—or both—of them has lost so much testosterone that their libido is dead and sex is no long part of the relationship.

Most men don't have the communication skills to address and resolve—or at least improve—their sexual performance issues. If they try to discuss it with a doctor, they can feel defensive and angry. Plus, talking about these issues is embarrassing, which makes it extraordinarily hard to face these problems and, thus, find solutions.

The Typical Relationship Dynamic

In this part of the chapter, I explain the emotional processes that can lead to the physical difficulties you're having in terms of sexual performance and how to talk about them. We encourage you to experiment with recommended strategies to solve your sexual performance issues such as premature ejaculation or absent or inadequate erections.

Premature ejaculation can be due to *performance anxiety*.

Premature ejaculation can be due to *performance anxiety*. You may worry about having adequate or enduring erections, so you rush to the end in order to successfully finish before you lose your erection. The problem with this scenario is that it completely ignores the impact on your partner. Where was she in the process? Was she satisfied? Was she finished? Is she happy, or did you simply take care of yourself? How you answer these questions speaks to the balance between your ego and your self-image and your intimacy with your mate. Are you scoring points? Are you keeping a record of any sort? Does it even matter that she's there?

Women feel wounded and unsexy and undesirable if you approach sex from the objectification perspective. They say they feel used, hurt, and angry—not a good situation for improving sexual performance or intimacy. Neither of you ends up happy.

Some men may have pictured themselves as sexual athletes and wonder stars, but now something's wrong. They're typically open to exploring issues like their blood pressure, their cardiac issues, their age, or any other "thing" that could be the root of the problem. Yes, they may feel sad and frustrated about "the situation," but they probably won't be too concerned if they can get a pill to take care of it.

Hopefully, as men age they'll learn that sex is not about keeping score, nor is it about finishing (having an orgasm). When they're young, sex is an opportunity to "get off" and to "keep score." But as men age, the finish line is less clearly defined, and they can mature into men who are focused on intimate expressions and satisfying their partner as a way of feeling sexual and masculine. They can learn that whether or not they achieve an orgasm themselves is somewhat irrelevant to a good and powerful sexual experience. They can learn that a good sex life is based on intimacy and sensual pleasure rather than an arbitrary yardstick of orgasms (by either partner). It's no longer is about the *score*; it's about the *experience*.

Sometimes the issue becomes more complex when there are physiologic issues that stem from aging. As discussed in the first part of this chapter, blood pressure, blood flow, sensory stimulation, stress levels, anxiety—particularly performance anxiety—become potential roadblocks on the road to sexual satisfaction and happiness.

Plus, it's really hard to talk about sexual problems with your partner, your physician, and perhaps your therapist. That's why good (or better) communication skills are key to any discussion of sexual problems.

Even if a man's partner is open to communication and wants to discuss his inadequate erections or premature ejaculation—and she's willing to experiment with helpful strategies—he will often begin to practice what therapists call "assumptive communications." He assumes he knows what she thinks and what she'll say, so he holds an imaginary conversation in his head without ever actually talking to her. Then he's disappointed, frustrated, and/or angry with her. This isn't the way to try to solve a sexual function problem. But, sadly, it's what many men do.

When a woman offers to discuss their issues, she can unintentionally trigger a defensive response in the man. He feels attacked and belittled, regardless of what she says. He can not only become defensive, but emotionally aggressive or hostile as well, which further exacerbates his dysfunction and makes him even less capable. Soon he starts to avoid sex altogether, afraid it will result in shame and frustration.

In such cases, many men start to fantasize about other women and other experiences, so they masturbate. If they can have a solid erection and a successful orgasm under these circumstances, then they're convinced that the problem is with their *partner*, not *themselves*. I'm sure you can see the frustration and the turmoil that results from this kind of thinking.

There are some behavioral interventions and strategies that can help. Foreplay, for example, can be developed into a behavior pattern. Arouse yourselves through conversation, teasing, stroking, and then pause. Relax and repeat as needed. The goal is to increase your stamina and endurance. You want to get to the point of orgasm but then learn to wait, back off, and begin again. It's a difficult behavior to learn, but it can be fun to practice. The goal is to learn to delay ejaculating so that it's not premature. Developing this skill can make your performance much more satisfying to your partner.

After Dr. Maupin has addressed the physiological issues such as blood flow, cortisol and testosterone, and blood pressure, and stress and anxiety levels are adequately evaluated, the key to an improved sexual experience becomes practicing intimacy and new behaviors.

Communicate what you want and like, negotiate with your partner, and put the focus on being more intimate and less on the orgasm. Talk to one another about cuing and how you signal your desire. Discuss your wants and fantasies.

Earl and Judy came to my office full of frustration and anger because they never seemed to be on the same page when it came to having sex. They both wanted to be more sexually active, but they usually weren't aroused at the same time. I asked them to tell me about the cuing and the flirtation dance that they used. They both said "huh"? I realized that I needed to begin at the beginning and explain. This is what I told them:

I used to show a movie to my anthropology classes about a primitive tribe in Indonesia. In the movie, the unmarried girls walked past the boys who worked in the fields, and the camera showed a close-up of the boys' faces. Their eyes would open wide and their mouths would stretch into huge smiles, and their chests would puff up. Everyone could see what they were interested in!

We are the same way. We cue one another to signal interest and the desire to have sex with each other. The cues can be smiles, spoken words or phrases, or touches, but we send signals to our partner. If your partner says something like, "Would you like to come upstairs and brush my hair?" or "Come wash my back," then you know that's your cue. She's interested and available!

Every couple has such cues, but they aren't always conscious of them. When couples come to see me about their troubled sex lives, I want to have them consciously recognize the patterns they use to cue one another. If they can't do that, then we rehearse and practice things that won't embarrasses them and teach them to communicate with more openness and specificity about when they want to have sex. Sometimes it is as simple as saying, "I want to have sex with you. Are you interested?" But for most of us, it becomes a habituated dance. When we're listening to the same music, there's no problem. But when the music doesn't match, we need to solve this problem.

Sometimes the key to cuing is simple: match your breathing patterns while making eye contact, put your arms around each other, and sway slowly to create a sensory experience. The main point is to learn to talk to each other using any language that works—verbal or nonverbal. Then, if needed, seek help so you can learn to approach sex from a loving and intimate perspective, rather than using the orgasmic approach (AKA, "Wham, bam, thank you ma'am").

Remember that timing is critical. If your partner is in the middle of reading an absorbing book, is watching the championship game, or is packing the kids' lunches, ask if they're available for sex when they're finished. There's nothing wrong with saying, "When this is over, can we have sex?" Don't make the mistake of sending silent cues and hoping to catch their attention, and please don't demand that they interrupt what they're doing to take care of your needs. This is the dance of intimacy. It's not about selfishness or domination. Talk, talk, talk, cue and dance.

Brett's Counseling Method

Because the initial trigger for this complex problem of sexual performance and timing disparities is often physical, whenever a client comes in and complains about his relationship and sex life, I suggest he have a complete physical. Men often look for a relational cause and don't realize their problem could actually be physical. It's much easier for men to accept a physical cause to their emotional pain, so we look there first.

I recommend that he make an appointment to see Dr. Maupin. At the same time, his partner should also be evaluated so she can determine if testosterone is the cause of her sexual issues.

Dr. Maupin referred a patient-couple to me. Mary had lost interest in sex, and her husband, Brian, was angry because he'd been "cut off." When they'd first gone to see Dr. Maupin about Mary's lack of sex drive, Brian announced, "If you don't fix her, I'm done! I won't live my life without sex!" That put incredible pressure on Dr. Maupin and Mary, who by now had been successfully treated with pellets for HRT (hormone replacement therapy) and had regained her libido. But so much damage had been done by Brian's verbal abuse that things weren't the same for her sexually. This is when they came to see me for counseling to repair the damage to their relationship.

Over time, Brian came to understand that Mary's lack of responsiveness before she'd received the pellets wasn't because she rejected him. Instead, it was due to physiological issues that had been corrected. Knowing that, he became more amenable, courteous, and sweet to her. As his attitude changed, Mary was able to forgive him for threatening to abandon her, and they rediscovered both their affection and their desire for one another.

Collateral Damage

When things aren't going your way sexually, you might think it's because your partner either doesn't desire you anymore or doesn't satisfy you in the ways you always imagined your sex life would—and should—be. You may not think in terms of your own performance; your own arousability, desirability, or capacity to hold an erection; or your ability to stimulate, encourage, and satisfy her needs. Men tend to be a bit selfish in this respect and simply ask, "Is it good for me?"

I counseled a couple, Harry and Ann, who couldn't get past Harry's paranoia. He thought Ann wasn't interested in him anymore and that she was going outside their marriage for sexual satisfaction. Ann's response was simple: "I don't like sex anymore, and I'm not going to fake it. I'm done."

Because we'd reached a roadblock in our discussions, I sent them both to Dr. Maupin, who interviewed them together for nearly two hours. Their blood work, combined with their individual responses in their questionnaires, showed that they both had low T, which could be interfering with their sex life.

Dr. Maupin directed her comments to Ann first. She listened without comment, but Dr. Maupin had the feeling that Ann wouldn't be open to taking testosterone herself as an answer to their problems. Then it was Harry's turn. He also listened but seemed to reject the idea that he might be part of the problem.

When asked about the quality of his erections and the length of time it took him to complete his "task," a funny thing happened. Ann moved her chair slightly behind Harry and started making hand signals to Dr. Maupin to indicate that Harry was not accurately describing his erections!

That opened the door to true communication. Yes, Ann had lost her desire for sex but was willing to work together to find a solution, as long as there was something in it for her. However, Harry's low level of testosterone had made intercourse more like work, and since there was no payoff for her, she had chosen to abstain.

Now that their shared physical issues were out on the table, they both agreed to take testosterone replacement with pellets. Voila! They didn't need counseling anymore. The problem was fixed.

Look in the Mirror

It's very hard for men to think about sex objectively because sex is so central to our self-esteem and our sense of masculinity. The following is an example of how couples can find themselves at odds by misunderstanding each other's cues and "language." It's also an example of the necessity of being open with each other.

Bruce, a fifty-seven-year-old male, came to see me because he was thinking about divorcing his wife, Dottie. He was angry and hurt, and he wanted to escape a situation that had become intolerable. He felt hopeless and had no idea if the marriage could be fixed.

He was tired of not being touched or held, tired of asking his wife for sex and being refused. There were all kinds of reasons: "Not now, it's inconvenient"; or "The children are still awake"(even though the children were eighteen and twenty-two); or "Later, dear. I have to finish the laundry and get the Sunday School lesson ready for this weekend"; or the most hurtful, "You're fifty-seven years old, and it's time for that stuff to slow down."

Bruce swore he still loved his wife. They'd met in college and had been together for thirty-three years. They had a good life, were blessed with two wonderful kids, and were financially sound. But there was no passion, no interest in intimacy (which was his word for sex), and he didn't want to live without that. So he thought he should get a divorce.

I asked Bruce if he was open to bringing Dottie in for a few sessions. I told him it would be a safe place to talk about what was going on—where there would be some rules and a neutral filter to help them both understand what was being said and what was actually meant. I asked if he'd like to save his marriage if that was possible.

"Absolutely," he said. "But she has to change. I can't live like this anymore."

So, Dottie and Bruce came in together and, you'd never have guessed it, but Dottie didn't agree with Bruce's assessment at all. Her point of view was completely different, and she was shocked that he was thinking about divorcing her. She still loved him and was eager to share her perspective.

"Bruce is always talking about sex, but he never really seems to want it. He doesn't reach out for me or approach me when I'm available. It's as if he doesn't know when I'm ready for sex. I signal him—or I think I do—but he doesn't get my signals. He'll say, 'The ball game is still on and I'll be up in a few minutes', so I go to bed. He falls asleep on the couch, then wakes up and comes to bed around two or three in the morning.

"When we go out with friends or are in public, he says sexy things and acts like he can't wait to get me alone. He and his pals joke about sexual things and have a good time. But when we're alone, he picks up his book or turns on the TV, and all that he implied is forgotten.

"However, he seems to have a radar for when I'm *not* interested and approaches me then. If I reject his advances, he gets angry and hurt. He blames me for not loving him and for being a 'bitch.'

Sometimes, even though I'm not really interested, I say OK and go through the motions of satisfying him. He's smart enough to realize what's going on and gets angry afterward—but not at the moment.

"We don't fight a lot, but there's tension there, and we tend to avoid each other. I'd love to change that."

Next, I asked them each to describe their sex life so that their partner could hear what they thought. As is often the case, when we got to a place where they could hear each other without feeling attacked or blamed, they could concentrate on learning better communication skills.

I'm always amazed how infrequently people actually talk to their partners about their sexual desires and sexual satisfaction. They always seem to expect that "it" (meaning sex) is a natural behavior that everyone has and instinctively understands.

Nothing could be further from the truth. Sex *is* natural and instinctive; it's a human drive. But we don't all experience it the same way, and we don't all want the same things. Behaviors aren't universal. Sex is such a critical part of our lives and our relationships that we need to learn how to communicate openly about it.

We continued our discussions after they got the results from their physical checkups. It turned out that they had both lost enough testosterone that their libidos had been adversely impacted.

Dottie's testosterone was almost completely gone, which is why she didn't have a sex drive, was rarely orgasmic, and wasn't excited about having sex. Her responses to Bruce were biological, *not* relational. *She loved Bruce and wanted to make him happy but never felt the urge to be sexual. When she tried to respond to him, her body simply didn't work the way it once had. She thought it was a natural part of aging and that their sex lives were essentially over.*

Eventually, Bruce admitted that he, too, had lost some of the "feelings and urges" he'd once felt. Once he realized Dottie wasn't attacking his masculinity, rejecting him, or ridiculing his performance, he could say that he didn't feel like the man he used to be.

While Dr. Maupin worked on restoring their libidos and resolving their performance incapacities (desire, lubrication, erections, etc.), we worked on improving communication and understanding skills.

They were surprised when I suggested we talk about the accommodations and cuing methods they'd developed as their libidos waned. They needed to be aware of these things and to learn to talk about them, so they could use different strategies and learn to love each other in ways that met the full spectrum of their needs and desires. They had to be willing to take some risks and to be honest with themselves and each other about who they were and what they wanted in their lives and their relationship.

Communication—The Key to Emotional Healing

Many couples need counseling. Dr. Maupin asserts that everybody needs a lawyer, a doctor, *and* a therapist! Her point is that people seem willing to call a doctor or lawyer when they need them but are often embarrassed to go to a counselor. They shouldn't be.

Counselors can help you improve your communication skills and make it possible to reframe and repair many of the wounds in your relationships. The art of communication has two main rules that can improve your relationship:

- **Communicate about difficulties and expectations:** We all have different upbringings that influence how we feel about sex. You may assume that your spouse is just like you, and that she thinks and believes like you do. So you operate from that assumption, while never talking about your differences. That's your first mistake! It's vital to look at why you believe what you do, why your spouse has her/his beliefs, and then proceed from that point.

- **Social/cultural/religious issues affect sexual thinking and behavior:** We've all been raised in a culture that has lessons and values that we've internalized and that produced habits of thinking and reacting.

This internal compass is what Freud called the Super Ego. It's why we experience guilt and shame (control behaviors) when our id (the biological, instinctive part of our "self") tells us it wants that pretty girl in the corner, but our superego tells us that we aren't supposed to want her because she's the "wrong" color, religion, family, or whatever.

Our families, schools, and churches tell us what we should consider "right" or "normal." In turn, these beliefs dictate how we feel, how we express our feelings (or don't), whom we desire, and how we act in an effort to be acceptable to the group.

It's important to examine your family messages. What did you learn about sex? Are you supposed to color inside the box or reject that idea? What if you don't fit in because some part of you is unacceptable to your family/group (transgender, homosexual, multiple partners, some other "wrong" behavior)? How do you present yourself to the world at large and to your partners as a sexual being? How do you function within relationships and experience trust and intimacy, while managing to avoid shame and rejection?

We all have to answer these questions for ourselves and must find a partner who shares our answers or is open to some level of difference. If not, there will be major problems in our relationship. If you want a happy and sexually satisfying marriage, it's vital to discuss your point of view, preferably before you marry. But it's never too late.

When I met Jack and Joann, I immediately thought they'd been attracted to their partner's personality type. Both were outgoing and funny and, despite their sexual problems, they seemed well suited to each other. But they'd been raised with completely different ideas about sex.

In the beginning of their relationship, their sex life seemed excellent, but after marriage, some weird things happened. Jack was no longer interested in sex; but now that Joann had finally gotten past the long drought of avoiding premarital sex—except with Jack—she was ready to roll! But no matter what she did (wore sexy nightwear, carried out daring scenarios like sex in the hot tub), none of it did a bit of good. Once they were married, Jack had lost his interest in having sex.

When they came to me, they'd been married thirty years. Their perspectives couldn't have been more different. Jack couldn't figure out what he was doing in my office, and Joann was extremely angry. She said that for the first ten years, she'd thought the problem was her; then for the next ten years, she thought it was him (was he gay?). After that, she gave up because by then her testosterone was falling. But when she got her T back to normal by taking pellets in her late forties, the sex problem resurfaced. They probably hadn't had sex more than one hundred times in thirty years.

We talked about what they'd learned about sex in their childhood homes. Joann's parents had loved each other more than they loved her, and they obviously touched and had sex. But otherwise, they weren't in sync. She had hoped her marriage to someone "like her" would be different, but she never considered she might not be desired, touched, or pursued.

Jack's upbringing was different. His mother was the primary parent, and she beat into his head that women who had sex with you were "whores," but women you marry were to be put on a pedestal. As a result, he put on the full-court press in college, ripe with one-night stands, but then slammed on the brakes after marriage.

Going through counseling, in addition to both of them taking testosterone pellets, helped this couple lose the anger and hostility that had plagued their marriage. The testosterone helped create the desire to overcome their preconceived attitudes that they had learned in their childhoods.

Self-image and Confidence

Our self-image is first formed through our interactions with our mothers. We study when they frown, smile, or meet our needs as infants, and this is how we draw conclusions about our own worth and attractiveness. As our world expands beyond our mothers, we try to get other people to respond to us, too. We want to invite and then control those responses, which provides another building block to developing our self-image. As teens and adults, we move beyond our families and out into the world, constantly seeking reactions and responses from others.

Do we create an image or a false self that we put out for public consumption? Can we reserve a separate image that we offer only to our intimates? Finally, do we have a private image we keep just for ourselves?

The answer to all these questions is "yes"! We all do it. And we continually monitor how it's working as we shift between our false selves and our restricted selves, seeking to gratify our needs, while being both safe and successful within our own segment of society.

In relationships, we dance between self-images—both our own self-image and those of our intimates.

In relationships, we dance between self-images—both our own self-image and those of our intimates. When I speak of *intimacy*, I'm referring to a condition where we remove as many of our masks as we feel safe in removing, so the other will experience us almost as we experience ourselves. This is the art form—the dance, if you will—of relationships.

Envision a series of concentric rings that continually expand and contract around a central nugget. That nugget is our self-image, and the fluctuating rings represent our interactions with others. Nonverbal communication leads us to sense if others are happy with us and if we are safe with them. When we sense that others find us attractive, desirable, enjoyable, and/or acceptable, we feel safe and can take the risk of removing our masks. This is necessary for intimacy, and intimacy makes sex much more satisfying and important in our lives.

When we're in a relationship, we're subconsciously—but acutely—aware of our partner's feelings. Their feelings are actually reflections of our own self-image. Our partner is simply serving as a mirror. When they're happy, we feel handsome or beautiful. If they don't like what we're doing or saying—or if they're angry—we feel ugly and unwanted. This is why partners of depressed people often become depressed themselves. They mirror the other.

So, our partner's mood and self-esteem can dictate how desirable we feel. In part, that explains why some stray outside marriage when their partner is sick, depressed, or angry about something. It breaks our self-esteem, and when our self-esteem is broken, we look for someone else to make us feel wanted, handsome, funny, or whatever we desire. Therefore, it's extremely important to keep yourself and your spouse happy and to preserve your own self-image—so you can preserve the marriage! Whatever you do for your partner comes back to you in spades in the bedroom!

Advertising Kills Confidence

We don't live in cookie-cutter bodies or have cookie-cutter personalities. We're all different. Each one of us is unique. And we should be. But that's not what advertising presents. Daily—hourly—we're bombarded with advertising messages that drive us to want to look and act like something we're not. And it's usually unattainable. Those messages destroy our self-image and sexual confidence.

To combat the destructive messages of advertising, you must find and nurture the things you love about yourself and your partner and say them out loud. Tell your lover that she's beautiful or that he's handsome. Let them know that you desire them sexually. Say it. Show it! This is what makes you turn off the TV, put down the phone, and satisfy your deepest need—to be known, accepted, and wanted for who you are.

Sexual Fantasies

It's always interesting to hear someone say, "I don't fantasize," especially about sex. I wonder if that's true or if they're simply unwilling to risk telling someone else about their sexual fantasies.

Testosterone is normally a necessary ingredient for men to fantasize about sex. So if fantasy is missing, you may be low on T. If your testosterone is adequate, then I contend that you can fantasize about the sex you want, the sex you have, or the sex you may never have but love to think about.

Sharing your fantasies with your significant other can lead to great things and can increase intimacy. But it's also a risk, so introduce this idea gradually. What's the risk? Your loved one could potentially reject you because they think you are "sick" and "disgusting" to dream up these fantasies. Do you want to take that risk? Or is it better to keep that part of yourself to yourself?

I love British comedy because those stiff-upper-lip guys have no problem donning dresses or wearing only an apron (think Benny Hill or Monty Python) as they act out their fantasies on film or stage. "Pretending" or role playing is one way to express fantasy, and it can be fun to do with a willing partner. It might just break through the predictability and boredom created by a lifetime of sex with the same person. Why not?

Now back to Dr. Maupin and some unusual situations surrounding testosterone replacement.

CHAPTER 7

Special Circumstances and Treatments

I've used all forms of testosterone replacement in my practice. As medical evidence and my own clinical experience have developed over time, I've reached the conclusion that, in most circumstances, the best option is to use bioidentical testosterone pellets to replace testosterone in the men who need it. However, this isn't always an option.

In this chapter, I address the unique circumstances in which pellets may not be the best form of delivery. Hormone replacement is complex. It takes a medical degree and extensive knowledge to determine who can and can't use testosterone and which form is the safest, most effective treatment for each individual. The type of T replacement that is best may change as a man ages, so we often change his T treatment over time.

When a Man Is Not Yet Ready for Testosterone Pellets

> **Even though they may have mild to moderate symptoms of low T, some men aren't ready to replace their testosterone with subcutaneous pellets.**

Even though they may have mild to moderate symptoms of low T, some men aren't ready to replace their testosterone with subcutaneous pellets. It's relatively easy to care for men over age fifty who have a total testosterone below 400 ng/dl, a free testosterone below

129 ng/ml, and symptoms of testosterone deficiency. Older men often need testosterone pellets to completely replace their testosterone production. But it's a completely different situation when a young man has borderline low T and mild symptoms but needs more testosterone to feel well. In these cases, the best treatment plan is to *stimulate the production of his own naturally produced testosterone*, rather than shut down his whole system and replace all his testosterone. (If you're still producing testosterone on your own—even if it isn't enough—and we give you additional testosterone, your system will stop producing its own testosterone and will rely totally on what we give you.)

If you don't yet need complete T replacement, you might be a good candidate for *testosterone stimulation therapy*. This treatment is best for men younger than fifty who want to maintain their fertility and men who have elevated estrogen levels, low thyroid, or adrenal insufficiency. A complete endocrine workup will be needed to determine the cause of the deficiency before a creative medical treatment plan can be developed to restart testosterone production by the testes.

Traumatic Brain Injury and Other Trauma

Sometimes a man's testes are fully functional and capable of making testosterone, but if there's no stimulation from the pituitary gland, the results are very low T levels. The pituitary gland, located in the brain, secretes hormones into the bloodstream, some of which impact the male reproductive organs. The hormones FSH and LH stimulate the production of both sperm and testosterone in the testes. If these hormones are low, then the testes don't get the message to make more testosterone.

We often see this in men with post-traumatic brain injury and/or PTSD. PTSD is caused, among other things, by multiple concussions. These types of traumas can cause damage to the pituitary gland and hypothalamus, which halts FSH and LH production. Perfectly normal testes won't work if they aren't pushed by FSH and LH to make testosterone.

Contact sports, auto accidents, brain surgery, and radiation to the brain can produce similar results. When the pituitary is missing or has been radiated, stimulating the testes may not work, but it's still worth a try.

The treatment is to give these men a pituitary hormone called HCG (human chorionic gonadotropin) to stimulate the testes. HCG mimics the stimulatory hormone LH, and adding this hormone can fool the testes into making more testosterone.

If HCG stimulation doesn't work, we prescribe Clomid® (clomiphene citrate), an oral medication that also stimulates the production of LH and FSH. However, it has side effects, such as developing man boobs (gynecomastia).

In young men, Clomid® works well to increase both testosterone levels and sperm production. However, in my experience, Clomid® and HCG treatments are rarely effective in men over fifty.

Brian was only thirty-two years old, but he'd been in three auto accidents in ten years. He'd sustained head trauma in each accident and had lost consciousness. In his first visit with me, he said that after the third accident, he felt different. He'd lost all interest in sex, gained weight, and felt completely fatigued no matter how much sleep he got. Brian had heard me speak on a local radio show about how head injuries can cause TDS. He said he knew I was talking about him!

He'd consulted neurologists and endocrinologists right after his last accident, but they reassured him that he was "normal." He knew he wasn't.

Although I don't usually consult with men this young, I agreed to do so because his two pituitary hormones were very low, and his total testosterone was very low as well. He was operating in a sixty-year-old body at the age of thirty-two because his pituitary gland had been damaged in the accidents. The only evidence of this damage was his low FSH/LH and low testosterone levels.

Brian's testes were fine, but they weren't being stimulated by the hormones from the brain. So he didn't need testosterone pellets—just stimulation of the testes. So far there's no method of "fixing" this brain injury, so we had to do a work-around to stimulate the testes so he could make his own testosterone. He preferred this solution, rather than using testosterone replacement the rest of his life.

I prescribed HCG subcutaneous shots three times per week to mimic LH and stimulate the testes. I also ordered two supplements to provide the building blocks of testosterone—pregnenolone and DHEA. It took several months, but Brian's total T and free T returned to normal for a thirty-year-old. Over time, we adjusted the number of HCG shots he took per week until he felt completely better.

Although he was young, Brian needed testosterone stimulation to feel normal and be healthy now. Sometime in the future, he'll need testosterone pellets, but for now he has the gift of feeling normal!

HCG Protocol:

- HCG is given in the form of subcutaneous injections or in sublingual (under-the-tongue) tablets. These hormones have a roughly 50 percent chance of restarting testosterone production.

- If HCG doesn't work, then it's possible that the testes are too old or abnormal. In that case, the only course of treatment is to replace testosterone with T pellets, no matter what the man's age is.

Clomid® Protocol:

- Clomid® stimulates the pituitary to make testosterone by increasing LH and FSH, which eventually improves sperm and testosterone production.

- Young men with low LH and FSH need stimulatory hormones to make their testicles work more effectively, but they do not yet need to replace their testosterone with pellets.

My patients ask frequently if I could "give them a little testosterone," to add to what their bodies are producing. Unfortunately, this won't work. If I give them supplemental testosterone, their bodies will stop producing it altogether.

Trent was only twenty-nine when he first came to see me. He felt that even though he was young, he had all the symptoms of TDS. During our consultation, I learned that he'd survived several head-on auto accidents for which he'd been hospitalized with concussions. When I tested his blood work, his FSH and LH were low, which resulted in both low total T and free T levels.

He was 5 feet 10 inches tall, quite thin, and had very little muscle mass. I asked if he'd played football and he said he hadn't—soccer had been his sport.

"Can heading the ball cause brain damage?" he asked. "Because in college, that was my specialty."

In fact, it's now known that heading the ball does cause traumatic brain injury that may not be discovered for years. Trent had several reasons to have traumatic brain injury, and the more often the brain is traumatized, the more severe the injury can be.

I asked him about his physical symptoms, and told me in a wistful voice that until the second auto accident he'd had a muscled body.

"But it's gone now," he said.

His low muscle mass was confirmed by our InBody® machine, which found him to be normal weight, with a very low muscle mass and higher-than-healthy fat mass. He'd recently stopped working out with weights because "it didn't do any good."

Even though his loss of muscle bothered him, his most important issues were his inability to think and to be motivated to go to work. He was also concerned about how his erectile dysfunction would affect his relationship with his fiancé. He was depressed, and rightfully so. He had the symptoms of a sixty-year-old man.

We discussed his options, and I suggested that we begin by using HCG to stimulate his own testosterone production. I added the supplements that produce the building blocks that make testosterone: pregnenolone and DHEA. I offered him the option to take Clomid®, used primarily for infertility in men and women. The downside was that it had the side effects of increasing belly fat and could cause him to develop man boobs. I told him that if both treatments were unsuccessful in bringing his testosterone back to normal young, healthy levels, we'd replace his testosterone with T pellets.

At Trent's four-month follow-up consultation, he was a very different young man. His total T was now 800 ng/dl, and his free T level was 190 ng/dl. And voila! All his symptoms were gone! The insecurity, worry, and depression he'd expressed prior to taking HCG were gone and his life was back on track! In regard to the future, he may be able to continue this treatment until he is fifty-something, and the treatment will help him with fertility when he decides to start a family.

I learned this treatment for post-traumatic brain injury from Dr. Mark Gordon, founder and medical director of Millenium Healthcare®, in Los Angeles, CA. Without his training, I wouldn't have known about the transformative therapy that I offered Trent.

Men with Normal Total T and Low Free T

Men often make enough testosterone, but it's inactivated because they also make a large amount of estradiol and estrone. This results in low free T; to the affected man, it feels just like he's producing no T at all. That's because the active T—the free T that actually works at the cell level—is missing or too low.

Men often make enough testosterone, but it's inactivated because they also make a large amount of estradiol and estrone.

Every year, I see an increasing number of men who have low free T but normal *overall* total testosterone. The most obvious cause is obesity, particularly beer-belly obesity. The more fat you have around the middle, the less active testosterone you have.

We treat this with Arimidex®, which is effective only if a man decreases his alcohol and carbohydrate intake and increases his exercise as well. DIM, an over-the-counter supplement, also decreases estrone and increases free T, and we use Arimidex® and DIM together.

As men reach the age of forty, the flow of estrone increases, which causes total T and free T to decrease—or to "leak" out of the bucket. For many men, dihydroteststerone (DHT) leaks steadily increase with age, which lowers the total T present in their bloodstream.

Factors That Contribute to Making Estrogen and DHT From Testosterone:

- Lack of exercise
- Lack of muscle mass
- Obesity
- Alcohol consumption
- Diabetes and insulin resistance
- Genetics
- Environmental estrogens

When DHT is elevated, it uses up free T. When we block testosterone from converting into DHT, total T increases. Just remember that it's important that DHT doesn't go below 25 because you need it for sexual function and muscle development.

When DHT is elevated, I prescribe finasteride (Propecia®, Proscar®). A 5 mg dose taken every other day usually lowers DHT and elevates the free T. Further, it may prolong the time a man can wait before he needs T replacement. There's also saw palmetto, an over-the-counter supplement that acts to lower DHT, but it's not as effective as finasteride.

Men with Low Total T and Low Free T

When a man has the symptoms of low total T *and* low free T levels, there are a number of options to explore before we jump to replacing his testosterone, which is an all-or-nothing decision.

It's up to the man to decide if his symptoms are severe enough to warrant replacing his testosterone, or if he would like to try a different remedy to block testosterone conversion to estrogen and/or DHT. Doing so can buy him months or even years before he needs to replace his own T, but this course of treatment is not effective for everyone. Sometimes we have to replace testosterone regardless, in order to get the optimal free T level.

When Doug came to see me, he was a forty-five-year-old respiratory therapist who worked at one of the hospitals where I'd previously been on staff when I practiced OB/GYN. He presented to me with all the symptoms of TDS, although he'd visited three primary care doctors before he came to see me, complaining of the typical low T symptoms. Each doctor had tested only his total testosterone, and they all found that his total T was between 700 and 800 ng/ml. By any measure, his total T was normal, so every doctor told him he was imagining his symptoms. He almost didn't come to see me because he was quite stressed about not being believed about his lack of sex drive, depression, insomnia, and ED. It turns out that he actually had a very low free T—45 ng/ml (normal is > 129 ng/ml).

I told Doug I could replace his T to a very high level to bring his free T back into a normal young, healthy level; but I offered him another alternative to T pellets: a course of the medication Arimidex®. If all went well, this drug would stimulate the production of testosterone, lower his estrone level, and increase his free T level. Because he worked in the medical field, he'd heard about this drug being prescribed to women with breast cancer. I explained what it did for men, and he was happy to try this option, which was less expensive than T pellets.

Doug has been my patient for over ten years now, and he's never needed pellets. After taking Arimidex® for four months, his T rose to 1,100 pg/ml and his free T to 180-250 ng/dl. Great numbers! Sadly, this doesn't work most of the time for forty-five-year-olds, but Doug was a marathon runner and his exercise has kept his T production optimal for the last ten years. Now I see him only once a year to review his blood work and renew his prescription.

I began treating Lee when he was fifty-three. He knew me from my "past life" when I was an OB/GYN and delivered babies and did surgery at a hospital where he was a pharmacist. He'd heard from some of the doctors there that I had discovered a new treatment for men with low testosterone. He knew about all the FDA-approved treatments and that they didn't work and/or had many side effects. He'd come to see me to "check out the new treatment I found."

Lee was such a delightful man that I didn't expect his difficult medical history. He'd had a misdiagnosis of prostate cancer in his forties and had a complete prostatectomy. He found out after the surgery that no cancer had been found in his pathology. He wasn't angry or spiteful; he just wanted testosterone, but no one would give it to him with that prior cancer diagnosis.

After confirming that his diagnosis was incorrect and that he'd never had prostate cancer, we discussed his options. He could have T pellets to completely replace his testosterone, or he could take Arimidex® off label every other day to both stimulate the production of testosterone and free up the bound testosterone so he'd have more active T. I was leaning toward the conservative approach of just the Arimidex® because his total T production was excellent (800 ng/dl).

We chose the oral pill rather than T replacement, and I crossed my fingers that this would make a difference for Lee. Happily, it did! His free testosterone was well above the minimum free T of 129 ng/ml at the first four-month checkup, and his ED and fatigue symptoms had resolved.

It is now fifteen years later, and Lee has never needed testosterone replacement. He continues to take Arimidex® and he has normal lipids, and no other problems except low thyroid, which I also treat. His total and free testosterone levels have remained about

1,100/175. Lee is now sixty-three and still works full time. He sees me once a year for blood work and prescriptions.

When Testosterone Pellets Aren't an Option

After treating thousands of patients, I have prescribed other forms of testosterone to only a few men, and it boils down to two reasons.

Inability to Retain T Pellets

Pete is one of my favorite guy patients. For his first appointment, he rode up on a huge Harley with his wife riding a Harley of her own. He entered the office for his first consultation appointment wearing full leathers.

A huge man, both tall and wide, Pete had many medical problems that weren't immediately apparent. He had high cholesterol, high blood pressure, autoimmune disease, very low T, and very high estrogens. His growth hormone was quite low, even though he worked out for hours each day.

Pete needed testosterone for many reasons. But every time I injected the pellets into his hip, they worked their way out and were expelled to the surface. I changed every part of the protocol, but his body would not accept the pellets.

Pete felt so much better on the pellets and his lab values had improved, as did his cholesterol, blood pressure, and autoimmune disease. But I had to find another way to deliver his testosterone. We opted for testosterone injections.

I warned Pete that the DEPO®-Testosterone in the syringe wasn't a bioidentical compound and wouldn't be as effective on normalizing his lipids and blood sugar as the pellets were. But we had to do something. In the end, he did well with testosterone shots plus a statin, but he would have preferred to come in every six months for the pellets versus every two weeks for the injections.

Very few men have the time or patience to go to a doctor's office every two weeks for a shot of testosterone. If they can't take testosterone pellets and they don't want to spend their life in a doctor's office, what are they to do? If they want to inject themselves with testosterone, what's the big deal?

Very few men have the time or patience to go to a doctor's office every two weeks to get a shot of testosterone.

I don't allow my patients to inject themselves for this reason: guys who have no medical training rarely inject themselves accurately using a safe procedure. And even a firefighter with EMT training harmed himself very badly when he injected himself.

Tony was the patient of another doctor, who had a written a script for DEPO®-T for him to inject in his thigh every week. Tony was a firefighter and an EMT, so he should have been able to inject himself in a safe manner.

However, he cut corners one time and the outcome was disastrous. Tony didn't swab his thigh with alcohol before giving himself the injection, and his skin wasn't clean. When his thigh became swollen to twice its size, red, and hot, he returned to the doctor who'd written the script. The doctor immediately drained pus out of the thigh, but this was now a medical emergency. Tony was transferred to the hospital for emergency surgery and intravenous antibiotics. In the end, he lost six months of work, lost half of his thigh muscle, and couldn't perform his duties as a firefighter anymore. He now comes to me for testosterone pellets.

It is critical to have an expert medical person inject or insert anything that goes deeper than a subcutaneous shot (like insulin shots) into your body. Because of Tony's disaster, I never write a prescription for anyone to self-administer intramuscular shots unless he's a registered nurse or a doctor.

Excessive thinness

We talked about Dan earlier in chapter 3. He traveled a great distance to see me to treat his Parkinson's disease, but at his first visit, he was too thin to receive the necessary number of T pellets. Parkinson's had depleted his skeletal muscle mass, and he had very little muscle or fat left on his body. Fortunately, his wife was a retired registered nurse, and I trained her to give him testosterone injections every two weeks in hopes that the T would help him gain weight and stimulate his appetite.

Within six months, he'd gained enough body fat and muscle for us to insert all the T pellets he needed for six months. With that, his Parkinson's improved and his neurologist was able to do something he'd never done before—decrease a patient's Parkinson's medications. We had managed to get him to a healthy body composition to hold his pellets and avoid the bi-weekly shots.

Summary

For some men, long-acting T pellets are not the answer. In the cases of youth, extreme thinness, an "allergy" to T pellets that causes pellet expulsion, and men who have not yet fathered children, we have many other solutions.

Conclusion

I hope you found many things in this book to guide you to sustained health through testosterone replacement pellets. The solutions I've presented are diametrically opposed to the teachings of modern medicine. I advocate for *preventive* medicine versus *acute care* medicine. I replace the hormones that disappear as we age rather than treat the symptoms of a hormone deficit with multiple medications; and I use effective, inexpensive, naturally compounded hormones rather than expensive, FDA-approved synthetic hormones that are manufactured and promoted by the pharmaceutical industry.

I boldly oppose the typical way Americans approach aging because I've discovered a new way to treat and prevent illness with natural non-oral testosterone pellets. I'm engaged in a battle with our institutional systems that control how we practice medicine, among them, the federal government's regulatory agencies and the pharmaceutical and insurance industries that work to suppress the information we've offered you in this book. The fact is that testosterone replacement will make you healthier and will restore your energy and sex drive, as well as your muscular strength. You will live longer and happier for less cost, and the "powers that be" don't want you to know that.

> **Testosterone replacement will make you healthier and will restore your energy and sex drive, as well as your muscular strength.**

There is a multitude of new voices speaking up to tell the world that men don't have to get old and fragile as they age. We're raising our collective voices to get the attention of men who can think for themselves and who will fight for what they need to help them age with health and strength intact, and with healthy sexual function for all of their days.

In chapter 1, I told you about my near-death experience and that I now have a purpose for doing this work. It is my mission. This book is part of that mission. I want men and the women who love them—everywhere in the world—to learn about the miracles that can happen as we learn more and more about replacing lost hormones and apply that knowledge. Losing your testosterone is the first trigger in a cascade of losses that leads to a miserable and decrepit life as you age, and our current medical systems have chosen to ignore this truth.

We haven't imagined this problem or this solution. We who have embraced this method are trying to rock the boat and get the doctors and the institutions that make up the American health-care system to recognize that loss of testosterone is a real problem and that there's a workable solution to the problem. There are thousands and thousands of doctors who have joined together in groups to promote this message and to change the way that medicine is practiced in America. And yet, the American Medical Association doesn't recognize these doctors or legitimize their specialties. I belong to two such organizations of doctors, the Age Management Medicine Group and the American Academy of Anti-Aging Medicine, and we are on the forefront of medical change.

What we've learned is that we must treat one patient at a time. It's like the old Chinese adage that a journey of a thousand miles must begin with a single step. We want to be that single step for you. Come on this journey with us and catch the wave!

Find a doctor who embraces testosterone replacement therapy as a successful, proven way to prevent the diseases of aging that cripple so many of us under the present system. Use this text as your guidebook to determine if you're a candidate for hormone replacement and then find a doctor who will help you avoid the diseases of old age and their debilitating impact. You must take charge of your own health care.

My fervent wish is that you've gained direction from this book and have found hope, and that you'll use this information as you embark on your journey to save your quality of life! Testosterone replacement via pellets is the foundation of youthful aging. Now that you know that those in charge of traditional medicine have tried to direct us away from T replacement with a campaign of fear that is completely unfounded, don't let those unsupported fears frighten you away from finding your answer to healthier aging.

> **Testosterone replacement via pellets is the foundation of youthful aging.**

After treating thousands of patients for over sixteen years with testosterone pellets, I am even more passionate about the success of hormone replacement—and particularly about testosterone pellets—as the most effective, least expensive, and most positive way to fight or avoid the illnesses we used to identify as being part of the inevitable aging process.

APPENDIX A
Questions Men Ask

The Superiority of Testosterone Pellets

What Symptoms Do BioBalance Health® Testosterone Pellets Treat?

- ❑ Low libido
- ❑ Erectile dysfunction
- ❑ Decreased ejaculation
- ❑ New insomnia after age forty
- ❑ Fatigue
- ❑ Memory and thinking issues
- ❑ Muscle mass shrinkage
- ❑ Osteoporosis
- ❑ Loss of motivation
- ❑ New migraine headaches after age forty
- ❑ Arthritis and joint aches

- ❏ Aching all over
- ❏ Increased belly fat, a new "beer-belly"
- ❏ New anxiety attacks
- ❏ New depression after age forty
- ❏ Male breast development

Men who need T pellets will complain of at least three of these symptoms.

How do you determine that a man needs T pellets?

If a man has low total testosterone and low free T and he has the symptoms of low testosterone, then he needs medical treatment to replace or stimulate his total and free testosterone and to relieve his symptoms. Men over age fifty generally require T replacement with pellets, while younger men often can be treated with medications that stimulate their own testosterone production.

What is the normal young, healthy level of total and free testosterone?

The normal morning *total testosterone* blood level for healthy men between ages twenty and forty is 400 ng/dl and above. The normal morning blood level of *free testosterone* is greater than 129 pg/ml. We compare the blood levels of men of any age to the blood levels of young, healthy men between the ages of twenty and forty, which is called the T-score. It's the same way we evaluate bone-density tests for osteoporosis: we compare patients of all ages to a twenty-nine-year-old of the same sex.

Should I try another form of testosterone before I come to your office for T pellets?

No. There is no reason for you to try a method that will not bring you back to complete health before you receive BioBalance Health® pellets.

Who is *not* a good candidate for T pellets?
Men who have not finished fathering children and men under age forty—unless they've had trauma to their brain or testes—are not good candidates.

What causes testosterone deficiency in men?
Aging, head injuries, post-traumatic stress, testicular trauma or surgery, pelvic surgery, mumps, tuberculosis, radiation to the pelvis or brain, estrogen-like drugs, genetic illnesses (Klinefelter syndrome or hemochromatosis), and autoimmune diseases can all cause TDS. T pellets can replace the testosterone, but they may not be able to fix all the problems that are the cause of low T levels.

Which blood level is more important, the total T level or the free T level?
I use both blood levels to diagnose and monitor men's testosterone adequacy. The total T tells me if a man is producing testosterone and if his testes are intact and functioning. The free T level tells me how much of a man's testosterone is actually working, and it's the most accurate way to measure how a man's testosterone is making him feel.

What are T pellets made from?
T pellets are all natural and are formulated from yams that are made into powder. The testosterone is chemically extracted from the yams and compressed into a uniform size per mg dose.

Where are T pellets inserted in men?
There are two areas on a man's body that generally have enough fat for the T pellets to dissolve: the upper outer hip and the love handles.

Does the pellet insertion process hurt?
No. Before insertion, we inject a local anesthetic (lidocaine) in the fat where the pellets will be inserted. The man feels only the numbing shot.

How often does a man need T pellets?
T pellets should be inserted every four to six months, with most of them lasting six months. The first time pellets are inserted, they last a little less than that, so men come back five months after their first pellet insertion to review their follow-up blood work and for insertion of the second pellets.

What might cause a man to need T pellets more often than every six months?
If a man has a large body size, is extremely physically active, is on multiple drugs that speed up the metabolism of testosterone, or has side effects from sustained high levels of T (like erythrocytosis—high red blood counts), then he may require more frequent insertions.

Why do men need more pellets than women?
Men naturally make ten times as much testosterone as women and, therefore need a much higher level of T replacement to bring them back to normal blood levels. Women can't tolerate as much testosterone as men, so they must come in three times a year for pellets, in smaller doses, compared to two insertions per year of higher doses for men.

Do the pellets dissolve after six months or have to be removed?
T pellets are completely dissolved (absorbed by the body) after six to ten months.

How long will it take for my pellets to work?
It takes about three to five weeks to get the full effect of the first testosterone dose. With every subsequent insertion, symptoms are resolved faster. Men start feeling excellent after only a few days with subsequent insertions.

Why does BioBalance Health® exclusively use testosterone pellets for T replacement in men?
T pellets make men feel normal and young like they did in their thirties and forties, while avoiding common side effects produced by other forms of T, such as an overproduction of the oil glands that make the skin greasy and mood changes like anger. With pellets, there's no concern about a man forgetting to take a dose or two or overdosing himself with testosterone injections or patches that can be easily abused.

More importantly, pellets have very few side effects. Pellets don't cause liver damage like oral testosterone does or prostate enlargement and testicular scarring like DEPO®-testosterone shots. Pellets also maintain a relatively stable blood level that can adjust to exercise levels, which no other form of testosterone can provide. Pellets also rarely convert into estrogens like testosterone patches and topical gels do. T pellets are like a reservoir that provides a man a constant testosterone supply that increases with increased blood flow like stress or exercise.

Do I trust Dr. Maupin and BioBalance Health® T pellets enough to recommend it to my family and friends?
This is the most important question to ask a doctor: whether he or she would treat their own family member with the treatment you will receive. My answer is "yes!" My husband has been on T pellets since I started treating men. He has been on them for thirteen years. As a result, my husband looks younger and healthier than any of his friends who are not on T pellets. I also treat my friend and co-author Brett Newcomb and his wife, Phyllis, and they are healthier than they were eight years ago. Both are at their ideal weight, and they have had fewer health problems than other people their ages who aren't taking T pellets. I have been on pellets myself for sixteen years and have never been healthier or looked better!

Are all T pellets the same?
No. We use T pellets from only two pharmacies: College Pharmacy and Belmar Pharmacy. They make their pellets from pure yam powder that is *not* micronized. Other T pellet companies cut corners by using cheaper *micronized* T to make their pellets. These cause many side effects like baldness, excessive body hair, anger, bloating, weight gain, and impaired liver function.

Testosterone and Erectile Dysfunction

Will I still need my ED medicine after I get pellets?
Maybe. Most men find that they don't need additional medication for ED. However, if a man has vascular compromise from arteriosclerosis or diabetes, then it's possible that ED medicine in one form or another may be needed. We frequently find that the man's blood pressure medicine is contributing to the problem, and we advise our patients what type of blood pressure medication they can take that's least likely to cause ED. In any case, if ED meds are needed, they're generally used at a lower dose.

How will T pellets help my sex life?
T pellets bring back the desire and motivation to initiate and have sex, as well as restore sexual fantasies and erectile function. Testosterone is the hormone that stimulates nitric oxide production in the blood vessels of the pelvis and the penis itself, bringing back erectile function in men (who do not have vascular disease). T pellets not only increase the hardness of the erection but make it last longer. The pellets also improve the quality of orgasms. Ejaculation usually decreases in volume as men age, but testosterone can increase the amount of ejaculate in some men.

Will my penis get larger?
Yes. Testosterone is used to increase penis size. Most men notice that they have a larger penis both at rest and when they are erect.

Will my testicles shrink after I take testosterone pellets?
Yes. The testicles will shrink to some extent. Testicles normally shrink with age. As the pellets take over supplying testosterone, the testicles don't produce as much as usual, so they get smaller. The "shrinkage" caused by T pellets is not a permanent change, and there are medical methods to stimulate testicular size, although it's a cosmetic treatment only and does not affect the activity of the testicles in any way when a man is on testosterone pellets.

What if I take testosterone and don't get any help with my erections?
First, we rule out bad habits like smoking, drinking more than two drinks per day, drug use, amphetamine or diet pills, and consuming energy drinks with high caffeine doses. These type of drinks and habits decrease a man's chance of having satisfying sexual experiences. Some diseases and prescription drugs prevent effective erections, such as diabetes, heart disease, arteriosclerosis, COPD, lung disease, drugs for high blood pressure, and steroids.

We generally evaluate the blood vessel normalcy with a cardiac calcium score to rule out any damage to the blood vessels. Next, we switch some of the blood pressure drugs to less ED-producing drugs. Further, we address the use of multiple antidepressants or psychiatric drugs, which can compromise the positive effects of testosterone pellets. In the end, adding an ED drug to T pellets and changing habits and medications can restore erectile function to most of our patients.

What medications can cause ED?
There are a number of medications that contribute to ED. Blood pressure medications like lisinopril, diuretics (hydrochlorothiazide), amphetamines like ADD/ADHD medicine, diet pills, as well as beta blockers for heart and blood pressure, multiple psych drugs, and Propecia® or Proscar® (finasteride) in daily doses can cause ED.

Why are testosterone pellets better than Viagra® for ED?
Let me count the ways! Testosterone fixes the real problem—lack of testosterone that decreases libido and sexual response. Viagra® does not address sexual desire. Viagra® is simply treating the *symptom* of ED—the inability to dilate blood vessel and fill the penis with blood. It doesn't treat the other symptoms of low T. In some cases, we use both T pellets and Viagra®-like drugs. Testosterone pellets have fewer side effects than Viagra®.

Testosterone and Prostate Cancer

Does testosterone cause prostate cancer?
No. Ever since I was in medical school, doctors have been taught that T causes prostate cancer. However, in the last decade, this has been disproven by researchers around the world. It is *low testosterone* over the course of a number of years that causes prostate cancer. Dr. Abraham Morgantaler (author of *Testosterone for Life*) has proven that low testosterone rather than normal young, healthy levels contributes to prostate cancer.

Should a man who has had prostate cancer take bioidentical testosterone pellets?
After prostate cancer has been diagnosed, the cancer cells in the prostate are completely different from the benign prostate cells that were there before the cancer started. If prostate cancer is present or wasn't completely surgically removed, it's recommended that these men refrain from testosterone replacement. However, if a man has had prostate cancer that was completely removed surgically and he has negative nodes (i.e., doesn't have any more prostate cancer cells), then Dr. Abraham Morgantaler, associate clinical professor of urology at Harvard Medical School, believes that the patient and his doctor can choose whether to proceed with T replacement. If the cancer has metastasized, we don't advise T replacement in any form. If the prostate and nodes have been completely removed and there is no recurrence of the cancer within five years, then T pellets are allowed for men who will sign a high-risk waiver.

Can I get T pellets even if I have a high PSA?
The PSA test is a screening for prostate cancer that is reliable up to the age of fifty, after which it's difficult to interpret. BioBalance Health® no longer orders a PSA test on the standard blood tests for men over age fifty who are starting T pellets. As of May 2018, it's up to a man and his doctor to decide if he should get a PSA test. If a man has a high risk of prostate cancer (African-American men, those with a family history of prostate cancer, or those who have had an abnormal biopsy of prostate), then his primary care physician will recommend whether he needs a PSA test. After age sixty, the National Institute of Health doesn't recommend the test because the treatment for prostate cancer creates a higher risk than having prostate cancer.

What is a normal PSA test?
In the past, the standard guideline stated that a result less than 4.0 at any age was normal, and anything more than 4.0 triggered a prostate biopsy. We now know that the PSA test "normal" rises after age sixty, and after age fifty-five, the treatment is considered worse than the disease.

What, other than prostate cancer, can increase a PSA test?
There are many things that can falsely increase a man's PSA. These include sex and exercise within thirty-six hours of the blood test. Other things can cause false positives when there is no prostate disease: benign prostate enlargement, prostatitis (infection of the prostate), having a prostate exam within thirty-six hours of the PSA test, and taking the drug allopurinal for gout.

Can I take T pellets if I already have an enlarged prostate?
BioBalance Health® T pellets will usually shrink the prostate in the long run, but in the beginning (the first two months), there will be a brief prostate enlargement as the prostate adjusts to a higher testosterone level. There are exceptions to this rule, but this is our experience, and we often prescribe tamulosin for a few months until the prostate calms down.

Other Aspects of Testosterone

Obesity – How long will it take for my body composition to get back to lean normal?
Your body composition will change, but the rate of change depends on how obese you are at the beginning of T pellet treatment. Other factors that influence the change are how much you exercise, your diet, and how often you work out with weights. Without testosterone replacement, this transformation would not be possible after age fifty-five, even with the perfect diet and exercise. With T pellets, your efforts will result in a younger looking and functioning body.

What about over the counter testosterone?
The supplements you see advertised on TV and online *don't contain testosterone*. These misleading ads try to make you think you can get cheap testosterone without a prescription, but you can't! Testosterone is *never* sold over the counter. These products they're selling are nonprescription formulations of herbs or proteins that are backed by false promises. And they don't work.

Testosterone is a controlled substance, and it's treated just like codeine and other controlled substances by the Drug Enforcement Administration. Only doctors and nurse practitioners can order and prescribe testosterone. Don't waste your money on fake hormones—save your money for the real thing.

Remember: If it looks too good to be true, it is!

Can I stimulate my own testosterone to a normal young, healthy level?
For men with low testosterone who are younger than age fifty, sometimes exercise, diet, and weight loss can bring your own T back to normal levels. After the age of fifty, we don't have much luck and choose to replace testosterone if the total T and free T both are low.

Are any supplements adequate to increase T?
If you are under age fifty and make a good level of total T but your free T is low, then the supplement DIM (diindolylmethane) and arginine/ornithine protein mixtures can increase your free T level. If you're over age fifty, you should replace your T with pellets.

If I failed to feel better on supplements that promised higher T, will I fail on testosterone replacement?
Absolutely not! Most of the time, testosterone replacement succeeds in bringing men back to health. Supplements are categorically a failure.

Your Lifestyle: How It Affects the Success of T Pellet Treatment

What will alcohol, marijuana, and narcotic drugs do to my testosterone level?
If you smoke, drink, or use marijuana, you will use up the testosterone pellets more quickly. This happens because your liver is overactivated and will metabolize testosterone more quickly. Using marijuana increases a man's prolactin, the hormone that increases breast size in men and women. Prolactin not only decreases your T level, it decreases your sex drive, ejaculatory function, and sexual stamina. We advise you to stop using marijuana altogether and to decrease alcohol consumption if you want to take T pellets and feel their full effect.

Caveat: There are some new strains of medical marijuana that don't increase prolactin levels or decrease T, so the above advice may change in the future.

How T Pellets Influence the Diseases of Aging

If I have man boobs when I start T replacement, will I be cured of them with T pellets?
Most men convert more and more of their testosterone into estrogen every year. Man boobs are stimulated by estrogen production,

and belly fat makes estrogen out of T. We treat gynecomastia (man boobs) with T pellets combined with the medication Arimidex®. This usually resolves the issue in the first year of treatment.

If I have adult-onset diabetes, will testosterone help me with my sexual response?
Yes, in most cases. But it may not completely correct your erectile dysfunction. It depends on how long you've had diabetes, how well-controlled it's been, and how much damage there's been to your blood vessels before starting T pellets.

Many long-term diabetic patients require T pellets plus Viagra®, Cialis®, or Levitra®. For men who've had many years of diabetes—especially without good control of their blood sugar—the vessels in the pelvis will be damaged and will no longer be able to dilate anymore to bring the blood to the penis for an erection. In such cases, the only treatment that consistently works is injections into the penis at the time of intercourse or a penile implant. Testosterone replacement provides multiple benefits to control blood sugar, improve body composition, help with weight loss, and prevent further deterioration of the pelvic blood levels.

Will T pellets mitigate the severity of my Adult-Onset Diabetes?
T pellets help decrease the severity of your diabetes so that it can be controlled more easily. T pellets increase insulin sensitivity, which will decrease triglycerides and stabilize blood glucose. T pellets decrease weight and, therefore, improve the diabetic condition. And by losing weight and body fat, you'll decrease the amount of diabetic medication you need, and you'll feel better!

Do T pellets improve autoimmune diseases like psoriasis, multiple sclerosis, rheumatoid arthritis, and lupus?
Yes. T pellets are the only type of testosterone that actually lessens the severity of autoimmune diseases. Estrogen exacerbates autoimmune diseases, and testosterone makes them better. We often treat autoimmune diseases successfully with T pellets. We

advise patients to continue their autoimmune medications until they're much better. Then they can talk to their rheumatologist or neurologist about decreasing their autoimmune medications.

Does testosterone replacement help prevent Parkinson's disease and Alzheimer's disease?

Yes. Both diseases are more common in men with low T, and replacing T at the beginning of the disease—or even in high-risk patients before the disease starts—can delay the onset or slow the progress of both diseases.

Do current and former athletes need T replacement at an earlier age than other men?

In general, this is what I've experienced in my practice; however, the physiology behind it isn't clear. Pellets tend to improve the joint function, cartilage thickness, and muscle tone necessary to relieve the pain from joint damage from years of sports. T pellets are also the best method of replacing low testosterone due to head injuries from contact sports.

Does testosterone improve depression and anxiety?

Yes. Taking T pellets often improves mood. Depression that occurs for the first time after age fifty is the type of depression that's most successfully treated with T pellets. T pellets can also decrease the dose of antidepressants needed, which is significant because most antidepressants decrease libido.

Side Effects of Testosterone Pellets

Will I go bald if I take T pellets?

Testosterone alone is not the hormone that causes hair loss in men. Dihydrotestosterone (DHT), a by-product of testosterone, can cause hair loss, but the inherited sensitivity of the receptor sites in the hair follicles is what determines whether a person experiences hair loss when they make DHT from their T. The truth is that if you have the baldness gene, you'll go bald with or without testosterone replacement.

If I have high levels of red blood cells, how will T pellets affect this condition?

This is a concern for men who take testosterone, because adding testosterone can increase the red blood count in anyone. If there's an underlying condition that also elevates the blood count, then it's prudent to diagnose and treat that condition early on when treating with testosterone. We will still replace T pellets in men whose blood count is raised if they are compliant with the necessary regular blood donations.

Why is it dangerous to have a high red blood count?

Elevated concentrations of red blood cells cause sludging (thickening) of the blood and could cause clots to form. It also puts a strain on the heart! It's important that this condition is diagnosed and treated prior to, or early in, the T replacement process. We will stop your treatment if you have a H/H greater than 18.9/52.

What other inherited disease could require me to stop pellets or give blood?

Evaluation of elevated hematocrit (the percentage of your blood that is solid—red blood cells) and the ferritin level can identify two conditions that are dangerous: familial erythrocytosis (explained above) and hemochromatosis. Testosterone makes both of these inherited diseases worse because T causes a man to absorb more iron from his food than he can use.

In erythrocytosis, T stimulates the production of too many red blood cells, which causes sludging of the blood (thick blood) and stress on the heart.

If a man has a high ferritin level, then he may have hemochromatosis. This genetic disease is made worse with increased iron absorption. In hemochromatosis, the body stores extra iron in various tissues like the testicles, brain, and liver, and it can cause damage to those organs. Some men stop making T because of their iron deposits, damaging the testicles or pituitary gland.

The only way to get rid of the iron is to repeatedly remove blood under the care of a hematologist or gastrointestinal doctor until the iron level is lower and the tissues mobilize the iron they contain. Phlebotomy is the treatment for this disease, and if the blood is adequately removed, a man can still take testosterone.

APPENDIX B

Hormone Imbalances That Cause Symptoms of Aging

Male Symptom	Hormone Deficiency	Hormone Excess
Poor Libido	Testosterone	Estrone
Erectile Dysfunction	Testosterone	Estrone
Infrequent or Absent Ejaculation	Testosterone, Oxytocin	Estrone
Loss of Morning Erections	Testosterone	Estrone
Insomnia	Testosterone	Cortisol
Memory Problems	Testosterone, Thyroid	
Loss of Motivation	Testosterone	
New Migraine Headaches	Testosterone	Estrone
Decreased Muscle Mass / Strength	Testosterone	Cortisol
Joint Aches / Arthritis	Testosterone	
Fatigue	Testosterone, Thyroid	Cortisol
Poor Balance / Coordination	Testosterone, Coritsol	
Increased Belly Fat	Testosterone, Thyroid	Cortisol, Estrone
Ringing in the Ears	Testosterone	
Thinning Hair	Testosterone, Thyroid	Cortisol
Depression	Testosterone, Thyroid	
New Anxiety Attacks	Testosterone	

Male Symptom	Hormone Deficiency	Hormone Excess
Male Breast Development	Testosterone	Cortisol, Estrone
Decreased Height (Osteoporosis)	Testosterone	Cortisol
Coldness of the Body	Thyroid	
Swelling of the Body	Thyroid	Cortisol
Loss of Head Hair	Testosterone, Thyroid	Cortisol
Brittle Nails	Thyroid	
Abdominal Bloating	Thyroid	
Constipation	Thyroid	
Thinning Eyebrows	Thyroid	
Goiter	Thyroid	Thyroid
Low Blood Pressure and Pulse	Thyroid, Cortisol	
Dizziness	Cortisol	
Poor Immunity/ Frequent Infections	Testosterone	Cortisol
Exhausted in the Morning		Cortisol
Sleep Issues		Cortisol
Irritability	Testosterone	Cortisol
Hypoglycemia	Cortisol, Insulin	
I Stay Awake for Days	Manic	
Achiness All Over the Body	Cortisol	
More Fatigue Than Ever Before	Cortisol	

APPENDIX C
Dr. Maupin's Low-Carb Diet for Men

Dr. Maupin's eating plan was created for men over age forty who are struggling to lose weight, patients who are obese and/or have insulin resistance, and anyone with Adult-Onset Diabetes (AODM).

In this simple eating plan, you count only carbohydrates. You may eat any amount of other foods that you wish. This plan has proved successful as a fat-loss solution for over thirty years. In fact, I have eaten within the recommendations of this diet myself, since I was diagnosed with insulin resistance (pre-diabetes) at age twenty-one. This low-carb diet plan requires you to count only *carbohydrates*, not calories, and there is no need to weigh your food.

This low-carb diet plan requires you to count only carbohydrates, not calories, and there is no need to weigh your food.

Follow this eating plan until you reach your ideal weight. After that, follow it during the work week and eat as you like on weekends.

Here are the rules for Dr. Maupin's Low-Carb Diet:

- Eat six times per day.
- Eat all the fruits and vegetables you like, except no white potatoes or bananas.

- At each meal eat 25 grams or less of non-fruit or vegetable carbohydrates.
- Eat protein at each of your six feedings.
- Never eat carbohydrates without a protein.
- Fruit and vegetables must be fresh or frozen—no canned food!
- Drink two servings or less of caffeine (coffee, tea, or diet soda).
- Eliminate alcohol from your diet.
- Do not skip meals.
- Drink ten eight-ounce glasses of water or the equivalent per day.
- Take a daily vitamin—preferably, Smarty-Pants for Men.
- Exercise four or more hours per week

The components of a good breakfast are as follows:

- 2 boiled eggs
- 1 piece of lean ham
- 1 piece of toast (maximum of 19 grams of carbohydrate) with butter
- 1 serving of fruit or yogurt with fruit—no added sugar

OR

- Yogurt with blueberries
- 1 piece of toast with peanut butter (sugarless)

The Do's of Dr. Maupin's Low-Carb Diet

- You must eat plenty of proteins and good fats. Vegetarians who don't eat any animal products will have a hard time following this diet.
- Carry protein-rich food with you at all times. Obvious choices are unsalted nuts, cheese and thin crackers, Greek yogurt, cheese sticks, veggies with ranch dressing, apples and peanut butter, protein bars with less than 25 grams of carbohydrate, and protein shakes with less than 25 grams of carbohydrate.
- Stevia is the only sweetener you can use without sabotaging your diet.
- Meat is an excellent form of protein as long as you cut off the fat.
- Use healthy fats like avocado, olive oil, and coconut oil.
- Eat healthy cheeses for protein like ricotta cheese, cottage cheese, sour cream, cream cheese, crumbled blue cheese, Swiss cheese, and mozzarella cheese.
- Add nuts like pecans, cashews, peanuts, and sunflower seeds, and wild rice.
- Eat on a small plate so you don't feel deprived at the dinner table.
- Drink a full glass of water with each meal.

The Don'ts of Dr. Maupin's Low-Carb Diet

- No "low-fat" foods
- No alcohol
- No diet foods; fresh foods only

- No more than two caffeinated beverages per day
- No skipping meals (especially breakfast)
- No sugar, Splenda, Nutrasweet, or other sweeteners except stevia
- No honey, agave, or other sweets or syrups
- Don't cheat!

Avoid the Pitfalls of Following the Dr. M Eating Plan

- Weigh yourself no more than once a week
- Use our InBody® scale at BioBalance Health® to follow your progress (no more than once a week).
- Never leave your house without healthy food in your purse or briefcase.
- Make appointments with a friend, spouse or trainer to work out on a regular basis to keep you accountable—no cancellations allowed!

It will take two weeks of following this eating plan before you stop craving carbs. Just remember that you'll be healthy when you are at your ideal BMI. This diet is not forever. You'll be able to eat any carbohydrate after you reach your goal.

You may feel ill after following this eating plan for more than two weeks, so go slow and eat properly during the week! If you get stuck in your fat loss, BioBalance Health® has a very effective medical weight-loss program that uses medication to speed your progress while you follow this eating program.

APPENDIX D

How to Make Sure Your PSA Test Is Accurate

According to the National Institutes of Health (2018), men who are at low risk and who are over fifty-five do not need a PSA test because the treatment is more dangerous than the cancer at that age.

Timing of Your Blood Draw

For seventy-two hours before your PSA test, you must abstain from any sexual activity, including masturbation, and avoid exercise and any activity that causes your body temperature to rise (like driving long distances with the heat on or biking). You should not have a prostate exam for seventy-two hours before the blood test. Doing any of these things may cause your PSA to be falsely high.

Medications That Falsely Elevate the PSA

Allopurinol, a gout medication, is the most common medication that falsely elevates the PSA test. If you are taking this medication, make sure you tell your doctor and/or do not take it for three days before the test.

Directions for Follow-up PSA Tests

Please have your blood drawn two weeks before your next pellet insertion. Do not have your blood drawn right after pellets are inserted.

If we ask you to repeat your PSA test, we will get a more specific test that includes a "free PSA." The results will determine if you need to be evaluated by a urologist.

These instructions save men the pain and anxiety of prostate biopsies for false positive PSA tests.

Frequency of Testing

PSA tests are done once a year for men under fifty-five and for men who are at high risk for prostate cancer. An annual PSA test is generally covered by your insurance. For more frequent testing, the initial PSA must be abnormal or you must experience a new symptom related to the prostate.

Men who are at high risk are those who have already had prostate cancer; men whose fathers or grandfathers had prostate cancer and African-American men, all of whom are at high risk for prostate cancer.

About the Authors

Kathy Maupin, MD

Dr. Kathy Maupin has practiced obstetrics and gynecology for more than thirty years, and for more than sixteen years, she has specialized in hormone replacement for men and women using testosterone pellets.

She received bioidentical hormone replacement therapy herself after a hysterectomy at age forty-seven as a last-ditch attempt to save her health, her career, her family life, and her happiness. Dr. Maupin credits the treatment with saving her life. She now helps both men and women worldwide discover the importance and life-changing benefits of testosterone replacement.

In 2003, she founded BioBalance Health®, a medical practice to help women and men treat the symptoms of aging with bioidentical testosterone pellets, preventive medical treatment, dietary supplements, and exercise.

Dr. Maupin not only has a lifetime of experience in treating men and women medically, she also developed and successfully promoted legislation in the state of Missouri that benefits patients as well as doctors.

In 2015, she and co-author Brett Newcomb published their first book, *The Secret Female Hormone: How Testosterone Can Save Your Life,* in six countries.

Brett Newcomb, MA, LPC

Brett Newcomb has thirty-five years of experience in private practice as a family therapist. He has worked with Dr. Maupin for years to help her patients deal with the psychological and marital ramifications of hormone imbalance and the necessary adjustments that follow successful treatment.

Brett was also Teacher of the Year at Lafayette High School in Saint Louis, Missouri, and rose from adjunct professor of counseling to be worldwide director of the counseling program at Webster University in Saint Louis, Missouri. He has consulted with schools around the country and has been a workshop presenter for major international corporations.

How to find Dr. Maupin and BioBalance Health®

For more information on BioBalance Health® pellet therapy, go to www.biobalancehealth.com.

Follow us on Facebook at facebook.com/BioBalanceHealth

Follow us on twitter at twitter.com/DrKathyMaupin

See us on YouTube at youtube.com/BioBalanceHealthcast

Find us on iTunes at itunes.apple.com/us/podcast/biobalancehealths-podcast

See us on Instragram at instagram@BioBalanceHealth

Address in Saint Louis:
10800 Olive Boulevard
Saint Louis, MO 63141
Phone: (314) 993-0963

Address in Kansas City:
4400 Broadway
Kansas City, MO 64111
Phone: (816) 753-6552

CPSIA information can be obtained
at www.ICGtesting.com
Printed in the USA
BVHW042043050319
541706BV00040B/1729/P

9 781732 276758